I0708070

Customized Orthodontic Brackets through Additive Manufacturing

Additive manufacturing is transforming orthodontics by enabling the production of customized devices tailored to individual patients. This book explores the development, surface finishing, and clinical performance of customized orthodontic brackets produced through additive manufacturing (AM). It examines the challenges associated with achieving surfaces with sufficient smoothness, corrosion resistance, and long-term biocompatibility in patient-specific orthodontic devices. The book also presents original case study data, providing practical insights into surface topography, oxide film stability, and long-term performance of additively manufactured brackets in the oral environment. It is intended for academic researchers, graduate students, and professionals in orthodontics, biomaterials, additive manufacturing, dental materials science, surface engineering, and medical device development.

Features

- Discusses the aggressive oral environment and key corrosion drivers, including fluctuating pH, salivary ions, biofilms, and temperature effects on stainless steel brackets.
- Covers additive manufacturing technologies, including selective laser melting (SLM), direct metal laser sintering (DMLS), and electron beam melting (EBM) for orthodontic applications.
- Explains surface finishing methods critical for clinical viability, including electropolishing, mechanical tumbling, thermal post-processing, and protective coatings.
- Presents experimental investigations using microscopy, XPS, and EDS to characterize surface roughness and composition of AM versus conventional brackets.
- Explores how post-processing techniques such as rotary tumbling and electropolishing affect bracket performance, bacterial adhesion, and clinical reliability.

- Provides practical guidance on FDA regulatory pathways, including 510(k) considerations, risk management, and process validation.
- Offers one of the first dedicated books addressing the specialized intersection of orthodontic bracket design, additive manufacturing, surface engineering, and regulatory compliance, helping fill a significant gap in the current literature.

Elena Kostenko earned her first M.S. degree in Automated Systems Engineering in 2010, graduating with honors. She later pursued advanced training in medical device development, earning an M.S. in Industrial and Systems Engineering from North Carolina State University, also with honors. Since 2020, she has worked at CDB Corporation as a manufacturing engineer and project manager, supporting medical device design, manufacturing optimization, and regulatory activities. She has led medical device development projects, encompassing management and functional activities for orthodontic treatment-planning software implementation and its FDA 510(k) submission. She has authored scholarly work on nanotechnology in orthodontics, shape-memory alloys, and nanomedicine-based drug delivery systems. Her current research focuses on surface finishing and corrosion control of additively manufactured orthodontic brackets, with the goal of improving biocompatibility, clinical performance, and patient safety.

Customized Orthodontic Brackets through Additive Manufacturing

Surface Engineering, Corrosion Control, and Clinical Performance

Elena Kostenko

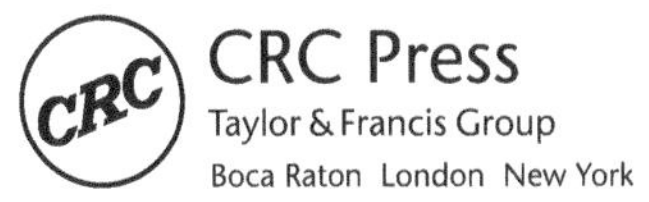

CRC Press
Taylor & Francis Group
Boca Raton London New York

CRC Press is an imprint of the
Taylor & Francis Group, an **informa** business

First edition published 2026
by CRC Press
2385 NW Executive Center Drive, Suite 320, Boca Raton FL 33431

and by CRC Press
4 Park Square, Milton Park, Abingdon, Oxon, OX14 4RN

CRC Press is an imprint of Taylor & Francis Group, LLC

ISBN: 978-1-041-30105-9 (hbk)
ISBN: 978-1-041-30109-7 (pbk)
ISBN: 978-1-003-77289-7 (ebk)

DOI: 10.1201/9781003772897

Typeset in Times
by Newgen Publishing UK

Dedicated with love to my sons Alexander and Evan, and to my father Oleg, whose spirit continues to guide me.

Contents

Preface

This book is the result of my research and professional journey at the intersection of engineering, materials science, and orthodontics. The rapid growth of additive manufacturing and digital dentistry inspired me to investigate how advanced finishing methods can transform the performance of customized orthodontic brackets.

My intention in writing this volume is to bridge engineering principles with clinical and regulatory realities. By integrating additive manufacturing technologies, microstructural analysis, surface finishing methods, corrosion assessment, and experimental validation, this book provides a unified framework for evaluating next-generation orthodontic brackets. Particular emphasis is placed on surface engineering strategies, especially electropolishing, and their role in achieving corrosion resistance, biocompatibility, and dimensional reliability in intraoral environments.

In addition to experimental investigations, this book addresses regulatory considerations essential for clinical translation, including FDA expectations for additively manufactured orthodontic devices, biocompatibility requirements, and process validation. By linking materials science with regulatory methodology, the work aims to support both innovation and patient safety.

This work was conducted at North Carolina State University, where I had the privilege of working under the guidance of Dr. Yuan-Shin Lee, whose encouragement, expertise, and thoughtful recommendations were invaluable throughout the course of this project. I am also grateful to Dr. Ching-Chang Ko (formerly at the UNC School of Dentistry) for his technical insights, and to Drs. Michael Kay, Jingyan Dong, and Harvey West for their valuable support and consultations. Special thanks are extended to Fred Stevie and Roberto Garcia for providing access to specialized equipment and for their generous technical assistance. Their contributions, along with the encouragement of my family and colleagues, have been instrumental in bringing this book to completion.

OpenAI's ChatGPT (5-series) was used exclusively as a language editing tool to improve readability and reader comprehension. This tool was used only for stylistic editing and refinement of English phrasing, as the author is a non-native English speaker. All technical content, interpretations, and analyses are the sole responsibility of the author.

Introduction

Orthodontic treatment has long relied on standardized appliances designed to serve a wide range of patients. While this approach has enabled predictable and efficient care for decades, it inherently assumes that a limited set of bracket geometries can adequately address the natural variability in tooth anatomy, enamel morphology, and biomechanical requirements encountered in clinical practice. As digital dentistry has matured, this assumption has increasingly been challenged. Advances in intraoral scanning, three-dimensional modeling, and computer-aided design have revealed the extent to which individual anatomical differences influence treatment efficiency, force delivery, and clinical outcomes.

Additive manufacturing (AM) has emerged as a key enabling technology in this transformation. Unlike conventional subtractive or forming methods, AM allows orthodontic brackets to be fabricated directly from digital designs, making it possible to encode patient-specific prescriptions, customized base curvature, and integrated mechanical features into a single component. Powder-bed fusion technologies, particularly laser-based systems, offer the resolution and material compatibility required for metallic orthodontic appliances, positioning AM as a practical pathway toward truly customized brackets.

However, the adoption of AM in orthodontics introduces challenges that extend beyond design freedom. The layer-by-layer fabrication process produces microstructural features, surface roughness, and residual stresses that differ fundamentally from those of conventionally manufactured stainless steel. In the oral environment, which is characterized by fluctuating pH, biofilm activity, mechanical loading, and fluoride exposure, these differences may influence corrosion behavior, biocompatibility, and long-term clinical reliability. As a result, the performance of an AM orthodontic bracket is governed not only by its geometry, but by the complex interaction between manufacturing parameters, microstructure, surface condition, and post-processing.

This book addresses these challenges by examining additively manufactured stainless-steel orthodontic brackets through a multidisciplinary lens. It integrates materials science, surface engineering, experimental characterization, and regulatory considerations to provide a comprehensive framework for evaluating AM brackets intended for intraoral use. Particular emphasis is placed on surface finishing, as surface condition plays a central role in friction,

DOI: 10.1201/9781003772897-1

plaque retention, corrosion resistance, and dimensional accuracy. Mechanical finishing and electropolishing are explored in depth, with experimental evidence demonstrating how each method influences surface topography, surface chemistry, and compliance with clinical and regulatory expectations.

Beyond technical performance, the book recognizes that successful clinical translation requires alignment with regulatory requirements. Additive manufacturing introduces process-dependent variability that must be addressed through validation, risk management, and biocompatibility assessment. Accordingly, the regulatory framework governing AM orthodontic brackets, including FDA expectations under the 510(k) pathway and relevant international standards, is examined alongside experimental findings.

By linking historical context, modern manufacturing technologies, surface engineering strategies, and regulatory methodology, this book aims to support researchers, engineers, clinicians, and regulatory professionals engaged in the development of next-generation orthodontic devices. Ultimately, it seeks to demonstrate that with appropriate design control, finishing, and validation, additive manufacturing can deliver customized orthodontic brackets that meet the same standards of safety, reliability, and clinical performance as traditional systems while expanding the possibilities of personalized orthodontic care.

History of Bracket Design and Materials 1

EVOLUTION OF ORTHODONTIC BRACKET DESIGN AND MATERIALS

The origins of orthodontic practice trace back to antiquity. Archaeological evidence suggests that ancient civilizations made rudimentary attempts at dental alignment using early orthodontic devices. In Egypt, archaeologists have discovered mummified remains with metal bands wrapped around individual teeth, often secured with catgut (a cord made from animal intestines), likely intended to apply pressure and manage spacing similar to primitive braces. Similar evidence appears in the Etruscan and Roman archaeological record, where teeth bound with gold wire have been found, interpreted as early ligature or alignment devices intended to preserve dental position in burial contexts. Though rudimentary and not comparable to modern orthodontic systems, these findings reflect an early appreciation that teeth could be guided or restrained, demonstrating that concern for dental harmony is not solely a product of modernity but spans millennia (Wikipedia, 2025; Bailey Orthodontics, 2025).

The formalization of orthodontics as a modern specialty began in the late nineteenth and early twentieth centuries with the pioneering work of Edward H. Angle. Angle introduced the first systematic classification of malocclusion and developed appliance systems based on standardized bracket design. His philosophy assumed that identical brackets for all teeth would simplify clinical practice and improve consistency – an idea that held tremendous influence throughout the twentieth century. Many contemporary appliance systems still echo Angle's principles, although now with greater biomechanical precision and material sophistication (Proffit et al., 2018).

While Angle's innovations shaped modern orthodontics, uniform bracket geometry could not fully account for natural variations in tooth morphology. This limitation spurred continued development of more adaptable systems. Throughout the mid-century, industrialization and new material science breakthroughs accelerated progress. Precious metals like gold and silver, valued historically for their corrosion resistance and malleability, gradually gave way to stainless steel. Introduced widely in orthodontics in the 1950s, stainless steel offered an optimal balance of strength, ductility, biocompatibility, and cost-effectiveness, enabling reliable mass production and predictable treatment outcomes. Over the following decades, aesthetic concerns further influenced appliance design, leading to the emergence of ceramic and polymer brackets – attractive alternatives for patients seeking subtle appliances, albeit sometimes with trade-offs in brittleness or friction. Titanium and nickel-titanium alloys later expanded clinical possibilities, introducing shape-memory behavior and superelasticity, which enabled lighter continuous forces and more comfortable treatment mechanics.

As dentistry entered the digital era, a profound paradigm shift occurred. The integration of intraoral scanning technologies, 3D digital modeling, and CAD/CAM workflows made it possible to visualize the dentition with remarkable precision. With digital design came the ability to fabricate brackets specifically tailored to individual teeth rather than relying on universal prescriptions. Patient-specific CAD/CAM bracket systems were developed, improving bracket fit, control, and indirect bonding accuracy. Indeed, verified clinical studies have shown that customized CAD/CAM-based appliances can enhance treatment efficiency and reduce finishing adjustments relative to traditional straight-wire approaches (Brown et al., 2015; Hegele et al., 2021).

These technological shifts align with the broader movement toward precision medicine and digital dentistry, where individualized treatment planning is emphasized. As 3D scanning, modeling, and additive manufacturing gain prominence, the orthodontics industry is rapidly evolving to offer customized, high-performance devices that respond to both clinical and anatomical variation. Recent work highlights the effectiveness of such approaches and their role in advancing orthodontic outcomes (Hegele et al., 2021).

Angling toward aesthetics and material science advances, the evolution of orthodontic brackets continued through the twentieth century. Initial systems used precious metals like gold and silver for corrosion resistance and malleability, but by the 1950s, stainless steel became the standard due to its strength, biocompatibility, and cost-effectiveness. Stainless steel enabled mass production and more predictable outcomes. Later, ceramic and plastic brackets emerged to satisfy aesthetic demands, though they often had limitations in strength and durability. Meanwhile, alloys like titanium and NiTi offered enhanced biocompatibility and elasticity, with shape-memory properties allowing gentle, continuous force application. Recent innovations include CAD/CAM-designed customized brackets and indirect bonding trays, enhancing clinical efficiency and bonding precision (Brown et al., 2015; Hegele et al., 2021). Additive manufacturing (AM), particularly selective laser melting (SLM) and direct metal laser sintering (DMLS), now offers the ability to tailor bracket geometry to individual anatomy and biomechanical requirements. These methods facilitate personalized treatment, reduce inventory waste, and create single-piece structures that integrate hooks, slots, and torque. However, these benefits introduce new concerns, especially regarding material microstructure, surface roughness, and corrosion behavior under intraoral conditions. Moreover, the integration of digital workflows in orthodontics, including 3D scanning, modeling, and printing, has supported the development of hybrid treatment planning systems that combine mechanical simulations with biologically driven design. The trend toward patient-specific orthodontics has significantly expanded over the last decade, positioning AM as a cornerstone of next-generation orthodontic appliance manufacturing.

BIOMECHANICS OF BRACKET–WIRE INTERACTION IN THE ERA OF CUSTOMIZATION

While brackets are small, they sit at the heart of orthodontic biomechanics. Each bracket acts as the interface between the archwire and the tooth. When an orthodontist engages a wire, they are not simply placing a piece of metal into a slot; they are creating a controlled system of forces and moments that determine how the tooth will move over time.

The basic principle is straightforward: a force applied at a distance from a tooth's center of resistance generates a moment that tends to rotate or tip the tooth. However, the ability to deliver this force precisely depends on several design parameters in the bracket–wire system:

- The slot dimension and tolerance influence how closely the archwire fits and how accurately torque and angulation are expressed.
- The bracket base shape affects bond layer thickness and therefore the effective location of the bracket relative to the tooth's center of resistance.

- The surface quality of the slot and the ligation method (elastic ligatures, steel ties, self-ligating clips) determine how much friction is present during sliding mechanics.

Traditional straight-wire systems assume that one set of bracket geometries can serve a wide range of dentitions. In reality, tooth anatomy, enamel contour, and clinical crown length vary significantly from patient to patient. These variations can lead to unintended rotations, torque expression differences, and variable bonding thicknesses. Clinicians often compensate with wire bending or bracket repositioning near the end of treatment.

Customized CAD/CAM and AM brackets are designed to reduce that need for compensation. By tailoring the base curvature to the patient's tooth surface and encoding the desired prescription in the 3D design, these systems aim to bring the tooth closer to its final position with fewer adjustments. Exploratory and clinical studies on CAD/CAM customized appliances suggest that such systems can maintain comparable treatment quality while potentially reducing overall chair time or the number of archwire changes (Brown et al., 2015).

In this context, additive manufacturing is not simply a new way to fabricate brackets; it is a way to fabricate different brackets whose geometry reflects biomechanical decisions made for a specific patient rather than for an average case. The chapters that follow explore how material behavior, corrosion, and surface finishing must all be understood and optimized for these customized devices to be clinically safe and reliable.

MATERIALS BACKGROUND: CONVENTIONAL AND ADDITIVELY MANUFACTURED STAINLESS STEEL

Stainless steel has been the mainstay material for orthodontic brackets for decades because it offers a useful balance of strength, ductility, and corrosion resistance in the oral environment. In conventional manufacturing, 316L stainless steel is produced through casting, hot working, and cold working steps that ultimately yield a relatively uniform, equiaxed grain structure. When brackets are machined from such material, they inherit this microstructure along with its well-characterized mechanical and corrosion properties (Xu et al., 2024).

Additive manufacturing, particularly laser powder-bed fusion (LPBF), builds 316L stainless steel in a very different way. A laser scans across a powder bed, locally melting and solidifying small regions in rapid succession. This process is repeated layer by layer to create the final part. The extremely high cooling rates and steep thermal gradients in LPBF lead to microstructures that are markedly different from wrought material. Typical features include fine cellular or dendritic sub-grains aligned with the build direction, as well as process-dependent porosity and lack-of-fusion defects (DebRoy et al., 2018).

Several comprehensive reviews of AM 316L stainless steel have highlighted how printing parameters (such as laser power, scan speed, hatch spacing, and layer thickness) influence density, residual stress, and microstructure, which in turn affect mechanical properties and corrosion resistance (Vukkum & Gupta, 2022). For orthodontic applications, this means that a bracket's performance is not determined only by its design but also by the specific processing window used to print it. Surface quality is particularly critical: partially fused powder particles and micro-pits on as-printed surfaces can serve as initiation sites for corrosion and biofilm formation if they are not adequately addressed by post-processing.

From a corrosion perspective, the stainless steel's protective chromium-rich oxide film must remain stable under cyclic pH, temperature, and microbial challenges in the mouth. Studies on LPBF 316L have shown that, when processed and finished appropriately, it can exhibit corrosion resistance comparable to or even better than conventional 316L. However, the same literature also emphasizes that defects and surface roughness can dramatically reduce that performance (Vukkum & Gupta, 2022; D'Andrea, 2023).

Taken together, these findings underscore why this book devotes significant attention to both surface finishing and corrosion: for additively manufactured brackets, these factors are central determinants of clinical reliability.

REFERENCES

Bailey Orthodontics. (2025). *The history of orthodontic devices: Where they came from and where they are today.* Retrieved from https://baileyortho dontics.com/the-history-of-orthodontic-devices/

Brown, M. W., Koroluk, L. D., Ko, C.-C., Zhang, K., Chen, M., & Nguyen, T. (2015). Effectiveness and efficiency of a CAD/CAM orthodontic bracket system. *American Journal of Orthodontics and Dentofacial Orthopedics, 148*(6), 1067–1074. https://doi.org/10.1016/j.ajodo.2015.07.029

D'Andrea, D. (2023). Additive manufacturing of AISI 316L stainless steel: A review. *Metals, 13*(8), 1370. https://doi.org/10.3390/met13081370

DebRoy, T., Wei, H. L., Zuback, J. S., Mukherjee, T., Elmer, J. W., Milewski, J. O., Beese, A. M., Wilson-Heid, A., De, A., & Zhang, W. (2018). Additive manufacturing of metallic components: Process, structure and properties. *Progress in Materials Science, 92*, 112–224. https://doi.org/10.1016/j.pmatsci.2017.10.001

Hegele, J., Seitz, L., Claussen, C., Baumert, U., Sabbagh, H., & Wichelhaus, A. (2021). Clinical effects with customized brackets and CAD/CAM technology: A prospective controlled study. *Progress in Orthodontics, 22*(1), 40. https://doi.org/10.1186/s40510-021-00386-0

Proffit, W. R., Fields, H. W., & Sarver, D. M. (2018). *Contemporary Orthodontics* (6th ed.). Elsevier/Mosby.

Vukkum, V. B., & Gupta, R. K. (2022). Review on corrosion performance of laser powder-bed fusion printed 316L stainless steel: Effect of processing parameters, manufacturing defects, post-processing, feedstock, and microstructure. *Materials & Design, 221*, 110874. https://doi.org/10.1016/j.matdes.2022.110874

Wikipedia Contributors. (2025, February). Dental braces. In Wikipedia, The Free Encyclopedia. Retrieved from https://en.wikipedia.org/wiki/Dental_braces

Xu, Y., Li, Y., Chen, T., Dong, C., Zhang, K., & Bao, X. (2024). A short review of medical-grade stainless steel: Corrosion resistance and novel techniques. *Journal of Materials Research and Technology, 29*, 2788–2798. https://doi.org/10.1016/j.jmrt.2024.01.240

Corrosion Behavior of Orthodontic Brackets in the Oral Environment

2

The oral environment poses a multifactorial threat to the structural and functional integrity of orthodontic devices. Constant exposure to fluctuating pH, enzymatic activity, temperature changes, microbial biofilms, and salivary electrolytes creates a chemically aggressive setting that fosters material degradation. Corrosion is therefore not only a theoretical risk but a clinically relevant process that may compromise treatment outcomes and patient safety (Fróis et al., 2023). Stainless steel remains the most widely used alloy for orthodontic brackets due to its balance of strength, formability, biocompatibility, and corrosion resistance, which is primarily attributed to the formation of a passive chromium oxide film. Nevertheless, if this passive layer is disrupted by mechanical wear, fluoride exposure, or thermal processing, then localized corrosion can occur.

In conventional manufacturing, 316L stainless steel is produced through casting, hot working, and cold working routes that generate a relatively uniform equiaxed microstructure and well-established corrosion performance. Additively manufactured (AM) stainless steel, however, exhibits a distinctly different metallurgical history. During selective laser melting or DMLS processing, rapid melting and solidification cycles create cellular or dendritic sub-grain structures, occasionally accompanied by porosity and partially fused powder particles. These microstructural variations influence corrosion behavior, particularly in chloride-rich saliva, where passive film stability is critical. Several studies report that as-built AM 316L displays good intergranular corrosion resistance (Laleh et al., 2019); however, high-temperature post-processing or heat-affected zones can modify the microstructure and increase susceptibility to localized corrosion mechanisms such as pitting and passive film breakdown (Laleh et al., 2020). Such findings highlight the importance of optimizing manufacturing and finishing parameters for clinical safety.

Different corrosion modes are relevant in orthodontics. Pitting corrosion is common in chloride-containing environments such as saliva. Crevice corrosion may develop beneath plaque deposits or adhesive remnants. Galvanic corrosion can occur when dissimilar alloys including stainless steel brackets and NiTi archwires are electrically coupled in saliva. Stress-corrosion cracking is a concern in AM components where tensile stresses and printing-induced residual stress may coexist (Karasz et al., 2021). Consequences include surface discoloration, reduced mechanical integrity, tie-wing fracture, and increased friction at the bracket–wire interface. Furthermore, measurable release of nickel and chromium ions under intraoral conditions has been demonstrated, with fluoride accelerating dissolution and surface degradation (Chantarawaratit & Yanisarapan, 2021; Mirhashemi et al., 2018). Even if ion concentrations remain within regulatory limits, hypersensitive patients may experience inflammatory or allergic reactions, making corrosion control a clinical necessity rather than merely an engineering concern.

Surface condition plays a central role in corrosion dynamics and biofilm retention. AM brackets often possess higher initial roughness due to layer-wise fabrication and partially fused powder. Rough or porous regions promote pit initiation and passive film instability (DelRio et al., 2023), while also facilitating the attachment of *Streptococcus mutans* (Fernandes et al., 2022), whose biofilms metabolize carbohydrates to organic acids, locally lowering pH and accelerating biocorrosion. Post-processing strategies, such as mechanical polishing, chempolishing, or electropolishing, can decrease roughness and improve corrosion resistance, although their effectiveness depends on bracket geometry – recessed zones may remain imperfectly polished and therefore more prone to corrosion (Tyagi et al., 2019; Eduok & Szpunar, 2020).

Figure 2.1 illustrates a comparative example. A conventional stainless-steel bracket reveals a smooth, homogenous surface conducive to passive film stability and lower plaque accumulation, whereas the as-printed AM bracket displays visible surface asperities and micro-particles. These irregularities represent potential nucleation sites for pits, biofilm adherence, and long-term degradation in the oral environment.

Because of these complexities, corrosion evaluation of orthodontic brackets should incorporate electrochemical techniques (e.g., potentiodynamic polarization and open-circuit potential), immersion tests in simulated saliva, and fluoride-exposure protocols that reflect clinical use conditions (ISO 10271; Eliades & Athanasiou, 2002). Beyond laboratory evaluation, longitudinal

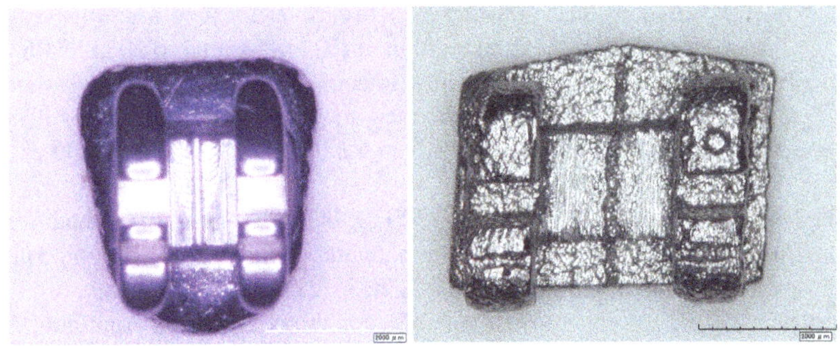

FIGURE 2.1 Comparison of bracket surface characteristics: traditional part (left) and additively manufactured part (right).

clinical performance data remain essential to understanding how corrosion affects treatment efficiency, device longevity, and patient health.

Ultimately, ensuring the safety and reliability of AM brackets requires a deep understanding of how printing parameters, heat treatment, microstructure, and finishing interact to control corrosion behavior. Regulatory bodies, including the FDA, require demonstration of corrosion resistance, mechanical durability, and biocompatibility for any intraoral metallic device submitted through the 510(k) pathway. As such, bridging the knowledge gap between AM metallurgy and orthodontic performance is fundamental for successful clinical adoption. The experimental chapters that follow assess the impact of finishing processes on the corrosion behavior of AM 316L stainless steel brackets, contributing evidence toward safer, more predictable next-generation orthodontic appliances.

REFERENCES

Chantarawaratit, P.-O., & Yanisarapan, T. (2021). Exposure to the oral environment enhances the corrosion of metal orthodontic appliances caused by fluoride-containing products: Cytotoxicity, metal ion release, and surface roughness. *American Journal of Orthodontics and Dentofacial Orthopedics, 160*(1), 101–112. https://doi.org/10.1016/j.ajodo.2020.03.035

DelRio, F. W., Khan, R. M., Heiden, M. J., Melia, M. A., Rodelas, J. M., & Schindelholz, E. J. (2023). Porosity, roughness, and passive film morphology influence the corrosion behavior of 316L stainless steel manufactured by laser powder bed fusion. *Journal of Manufacturing Processes, 103*, 654–662. https://doi.org/10.1016/j.jmapro.2023.07.062

Eduok, U., & Szpunar, J. A. (2020). In vitro corrosion studies of stainless-steel dental substrates during *Porphyromonas gingivalis* biofilm growth in artificial saliva solutions. *RSC Advances, 10*(52), 31280–31294. https://doi.org/10.1039/D0RA05500J

Eliades, T., & Athanasiou, A. E. (2002). In vivo aging of orthodontic alloys: Implications for corrosion potential, nickel release, and biocompatibility. *The Angle Orthodontist, 72*(3), 222–237.

Fernandes, R. B., Polo, A. B., Rocha, V. N., Vitral, R. W. F., Apolônio, A. C. M., & Campos, M. J. S. (2022). Influence of orthodontic brackets design and surface properties on the cariogenic *Streptococcus mutans* adhesion. *Saudi Dental Journal, 34*(4), 321–327. https://doi.org/10.1016/j.sdentj.2022.03.008

Fróis, A., Santos A. C., & Louro, C. S. (2023). Corrosion of fixed orthodontic appliances: Causes, concerns and mitigation strategies. *Metals, 13*(12), 1955. https://doi.org/10.3390/met13121955

International Organization for Standardization. (2020). *ISO 10271:2020 – Dentistry – Corrosion test methods for metallic materials.* ISO.

Karasz, E. K., Taylor, J. M., Autenrieth, D. M., Reu, P. L., Johnson, K., Melia, M. A., Noell, P., & Schindelholz, E. J. (2021). Measuring the residual stress and stress corrosion cracking susceptibility of additively manufactured 316L by ASTM G36-94. *Corrosion, 78*(1), 3–12. https://doi.org/10.5006/3894

Laleh, M., Hughes, A. E., Xu, W., Cizek, P., & Tan, M. Y. (2020). Unanticipated drastic decline in pitting corrosion resistance of additively manufactured 316L stainless steel after high-temperature post-processing. *Corrosion Science, 165*, 108412. https://doi.org/10.1016/j.corsci.2019.108412

Laleh, M., Hughes, A. E., Xu, W., Haghdadi, N., Wang, K., Cizek, P., Gibson, I., & Tan, M. Y. (2019). On the unusual intergranular corrosion resistance of 316L stainless steel additively manufactured by selective laser melting. *Corrosion Science, 161*, 108189. https://doi.org/10.1016/j.corsci.2019.108189

Mirhashemi, A. H., Jahangiri, S., & Kharrazifard, M. (2018). Release of nickel and chromium ions from orthodontic wires following the use of teeth-whitening mouthwashes. *Progress in Orthodontics, 19*, 4. https://doi.org/10.1186/s40510-018-0203-7

Tyagi, P., Goulet, T., Riso, C., Stephenson, R., Chuenprateep, N., Schlitzer, J., Benton, C., & Garcia-Moreno, F. (2019). Reducing the roughness of internal surface of an additive manufacturing produced 316 steel component by chempolishing and electropolishing. *Additive Manufacturing, 25*, 32–38. https://doi.org/10.1016/j.addma.2018.11.001

Additive Manufacturing Technologies and Microstructural Effects in Orthodontics

3

OVERVIEW OF METAL ADDITIVE MANUFACTURING PROCESSES FOR ORTHODONTICS

Powder-bed fusion (PBF) techniques dominate the additive manufacturing space for metallic orthodontic devices due to their high resolution, scalability, and suitability for medical-grade alloys. Their ability to fabricate complex geometries layer by layer enables the production of fully customized orthodontic brackets that can reflect patient-specific anatomies with minimal manual adjustment. Among metal AM technologies, the most widely used are Selective Laser Melting (SLM), Direct Metal Laser Sintering (DMLS), and Electron Beam Melting (EBM), each offering unique advantages, limitations, and surface characteristics relevant to intraoral performance (Vafadar et al., 2021).

DOI: 10.1201/9781003772897-4

SLM and DMLS are both laser-based powder-bed fusion techniques used to fabricate metal parts through selective melting of thin powder layers. In SLM, the powder is fully melted, resulting in dense parts with minimal porosity and good mechanical properties. In DMLS, depending on the energy input, the powder may undergo partial melting or solid-state sintering, which can produce components with varying density and microstructural uniformity. This variability directly affects fatigue resistance, corrosion behavior, and finishing outcomes (Wang et al., 2018; Vafadar et al., 2021). In orthodontic manufacturing, this distinction is non-trivial: even slight porosity differences may compound over time under cyclic mastication loads or during archwire sliding, influencing appliance durability.

EBM uses an electron beam under high vacuum to fuse the powder bed, enabling efficient processing of reactive alloys such as titanium and Ti–6Al–4V. The build chamber typically operates above 600 °C, leading to lower residual stresses and reduced warping risk compared to laser-based systems. However, the high thermal conditions combined with the vacuum environment generally result in rougher as-built surfaces, which require substantial finishing to meet intraoral smoothness and hygiene requirements (Fousova et al., 2018). These differences highlight that although multiple PBF systems can theoretically produce orthodontic brackets, SLM/DMLS currently offer the most practical pathway for high-detail stainless-steel orthodontic hardware.

In orthodontics, the clinical potential of metal AM includes:

- Custom-fit bracket base curvature conforming to individual tooth anatomy,
- Integrated mechanical features–torque, offset, hooks, and tie-wings built into a single print,
- On-demand production with reduced material waste, eliminating the need for large bracket inventories,
- Streamlined digital workflows from scan to bracket, facilitating remote fabrication and tele-orthodontic models.

Yet, the transition from research to widespread chairside adoption faces several engineering and biological challenges, including:

- High surface roughness affecting plaque accumulation, corrosion, and patient comfort,
- Residual stresses and thermal gradients leading to warping or crack initiation during service,
- Microstructural inhomogeneities and porosity influencing fatigue behavior, friction, and ionic release in saliva (Vukkum & Gupta, 2022).

The oral cavity presents a uniquely aggressive electrochemical environment. Variations in pH, enzymatic activity, temperature cycling, biofilm formation, and salivary ionic composition foster corrosion mechanisms capable of undermining device longevity. As a result, post-processing and surface finishing strategies are central to the clinical reliability of AM orthodontic brackets. Among finishing strategies, electropolishing consistently reduces as-printed roughness in AM 316L stainless steel, smooths asperities, and increases resistance to localized corrosion by improving passive film stability. Grinding and other mechanical finishing methods may produce comparable surface roughness improvements but typically involve greater bulk material removal, while passivation alone offers limited benefit without prior mechanical smoothing (Tyagi et al., 2020; Melia et al., 2020). Thermal treatments such as stress-relief annealing or hot isostatic pressing (HIP) can further reduce porosity and mitigate residual stresses, but excessive thermal exposure risks altering geometry or inducing carbide precipitation if improperly tuned.

PROCESS PARAMETERS, MICROSTRUCTURE, AND DEFECTS IN LPBF 316L

One of the defining characteristics of AM stainless steel arises from rapid thermal cycling during layer formation. This process generates columnar grains and cellular sub-grain structures, frequently aligned along the build direction, and creates heat-affected zones (HAZ) at layer interfaces that may be susceptible to sensitization or localized corrosion. These microstructural features contribute to anisotropic mechanical properties, meaning strength, ductility, and wear behavior may vary depending on print orientation (DebRoy et al., 2018). According to Vukkum & Gupta (2022), the interplay between powder morphology, energy density, and scan strategy influences not only porosity content, but also the chemical continuity of the passive film, showing direct links between printing conditions and corrosion outcomes.

LPBF processing involves interacting variables such as laser power, scan speed, hatch spacing, layer thickness, and beam diameter that determine melt-pool stability. Low energy density may cause lack-of-fusion porosity, whereas excessive heat input promotes keyholing and vaporization defects, degrading passive film chemistry and mechanical performance (DebRoy et al., 2018; Bose et al., 2018; D'Andrea, 2023). Because orthodontic brackets experience cyclic loading and frictional sliding forces, porosity-induced weaknesses are clinically significant. To ensure reliable bracket performance, > 99% density is recommended so components retain structural integrity during polishing and long-term use.

Microstructure also affects surface finish responsiveness. Coarse-scan strategies may generate rougher surfaces with unmelted particles, whereas optimized scanning improves homogeneity. Understanding this relationship is critical because the final mechanical and corrosion behavior of AM brackets is strongly dependent on both printing and finishing phases.

RESIDUAL STRESSES, HEAT TREATMENT, AND DIMENSIONAL ACCURACY

Residual stresses develop due to steep temperature gradients during melt-pool solidification and contraction. Without intervention, these stresses can cause distortion, warping, or microcracking, which is unacceptable for high-precision orthodontic brackets. Stress-relief heat treatments are therefore necessary, though they require optimization to balance stress reduction with preservation of mechanical properties and dimensional tolerance (DebRoy et al., 2018; Vukkum & Gupta, 2022).

Dimensional changes also occur during support removal, grinding, barrel finishing, and electropolishing, making tolerance control critical. Brackets require precise accuracy because minor dimensional shifts in slot height or width affect archwire fit, friction, and biomechanical force delivery. The later experimental chapters of this book analyze dimensional reduction after finishing, establishing offset guidelines for CAD modeling to ensure final clinical accuracy.

SURFACE TOPOGRAPHY AND THE "STAIR-STEP" EFFECT

Surface roughness is another central clinical concern. As-printed metal surfaces often retain partially fused powder particles and staircase artifacts from layer-based fabrication. These features increase friction with archwires, reduce sliding efficiency, and offer micro-depressions that harbor plaque and oral bacteria. Crevice formation promotes low-oxygen corrosion, while biofilm metabolism lowers local pH, accelerating passive film breakdown (DelRio et al., 2023). Multiple studies report that electropolishing significantly reduces surface roughness and improves corrosion resistance in additively manufactured stainless steel, enhancing surface smoothness and material stability (Tyagi et al., 2020). Still, recessed geometries under tie-wings may remain under-polished and continue to accumulate debris, highlighting the need for hybrid finishing approaches.

Beyond conventional mechanical and electrochemical polishing, advanced surface engineering strategies, including laser remelting, chemical passivation, nano-coatings, and multilayer barrier films, are under development to refine microtopography and enhance corrosion resistance in metallic biomaterials (Unune et al., 2022). With further improvement, these approaches may provide high-gloss, low-friction surfaces without excessive material removal, enabling brackets that combine biomechanical precision with durability in the oral environment.

As AM orthodontics evolves, it is increasingly clear that device performance is the combined result of printing conditions, microstructure formation, surface state, and post-processing. Emerging literature suggests that the corrosion resistance of LPBF 316L is intrinsically tied to porosity content and passive film morphology, with smoother surfaces delaying pitting initiation and improving breakdown potential (DelRio et al., 2023; Vukkum & Gupta, 2022). In this context, surface finishing is not merely cosmetic as it directly governs clinical reliability, hygiene, and biocompatibility. Future orthodontic workflows will likely depend on validated finishing protocols alongside real-time digital manufacturing, ensuring that printed brackets achieve the same standardized reliability expected from traditional stainless-steel systems.

REFERENCES

Bose, S., Ke, D., Sahasrabudhe, H., & Bandyopadhyay, A. (2018). Additive manufacturing of biomaterials. *Progress in Materials Science, 93*, 45–111. https://doi.org/10.1016/j.pmatsci.2017.08.003

D'Andrea, D. (2023). Additive manufacturing of AISI 316L stainless steel: A review. *Metals, 13*(8), 1370. https://doi.org/10.3390/met13081370

DebRoy, T., Wei, H. L., Zuback, J. S., Mukherjee, T., Elmer, J. W., Milewski, J. O., Beese, A. M., Wilson-Heid, A., De, A., & Zhang, W. (2018). Additive manufacturing of metallic components: Process, structure and properties. *Progress in Materials Science, 92,* 112–224. https://doi.org/10.1016/j.pmatsci.2017.10.001

DelRio, F. W., Khan, R. M., Heiden, M. J., Melia, M. A., Rodelas, J. M., & Schindelholz, E. J. (2023). Porosity, roughness, and passive film morphology influence the corrosion behavior of 316L stainless steel manufactured by laser powder bed fusion. *Journal of Manufacturing Processes, 103*, 654–662. https://doi.org/10.1016/j.jmapro.2023.07.062

Fousová, M., Vojtěch, D., Doubrava, K., Daniel, M., & Kneppo, J. (2018). Influence of inherent surface and internal defects on mechanical properties of additively manufactured Ti–6Al–4V alloy: Comparison between selective laser melting and electron beam melting. *Materials, 11*(4), 537. https://doi.org/10.3390/ma11040537

Melia, M. A., Duran, J. G., Koepke, J. R., Saiz, D. J., Jared, B. H., & Schindelholz, E. J. (2020). How build angle and post-processing impact roughness and corrosion of additively manufactured 316L stainless steel. *npj Materials Degradation, 4*, 21. https://doi.org/10.1038/s41529-020-00126-5

Tyagi, P., Brent, D., Saunders, T., Goulet, T., Riso, C., Klein, K., & García-Moreno, F. (2020). Roughness reduction of additively manufactured steel by electropolishing. *The International Journal of Advanced Manufacturing Technology, 106*, 1337–1344. https://doi.org/10.1007/s00 170-019-04720-z

Unune, D. R., Brown, G. R., & Reilly, G. C. (2022). Thermal-based surface modification techniques for enhancing the corrosion and wear resistance of metallic implants: A review. *Vacuum, 203*, 111298. https://doi.org/ 10.1016/j.vacuum.2022.111298

Vafadar, A., Guzzomi, F., Rassau, A., & Hayward, K. (2021). Advances in metal additive manufacturing: A review of common processes, industrial applications, and current challenges. *Applied Sciences, 11*(3), 1213. https://doi.org/10.3390/app11031213

Vukkum, V. B., & Gupta, R. K. (2022). Review on corrosion performance of laser powder-bed fusion printed 316L stainless steel: Effect of processing parameters, manufacturing defects, post-processing, feedstock, and microstructure. *Materials & Design, 221*, 110874. https://doi.org/ 10.1016/j.matdes.2022.110874

Wang, D., Wu, S., Yang, Y., Dou, W., Deng, S., Wang, Z., & Li, S. (2018). The effect of a scanning strategy on the residual stress of 316L steel parts fabricated by selective laser melting (SLM). *Materials, 11*(10), 1821. https://doi.org/10.3390/ma11101821

Surface Finishing Methods for Additively Manufactured Brackets

4

ELECTROPOLISHING

Electropolishing is an electrochemical process that selectively removes microscopic surface asperities by anodic dissolution in a controlled electrolyte environment. In AM stainless steel brackets, this technique can substantially reduce surface roughness (Ra) to values below 0.2 μm to minimize bacterial retention and plaque buildup.

Beyond surface smoothing, electropolishing improves aesthetic appearance and promotes the formation of a uniform, chromium-rich passive oxide film. This chemically stable surface layer enhances resistance to localized corrosion and ion release, thereby supporting long-term biocompatibility in the aggressive oral environment. Because material removal occurs at the atomic scale rather than through mechanical abrasion, electropolishing avoids the introduction of residual stresses or surface damage and is particularly well suited for intricate bracket geometries.

Nevertheless, electropolishing efficiency is strongly influenced by component geometry and surface accessibility. Regions such as deep undercuts, narrow grooves, or areas with limited electrolyte flow may experience

DOI: 10.1201/9781003772897-5

non-uniform current distribution, leading to uneven material removal. As a result, process parameters often require optimization, and in some cases, electropolishing may be combined with complementary finishing strategies to ensure consistent surface quality across all functional regions of the bracket (Tyagi et al., 2019; Melia et al., 2020).

MECHANICAL FINISHING

Mechanical polishing techniques, such as abrasive blasting, rotary tumbling, and vibratory polishing, are used to remove surface roughness and residual powder particles from additively manufactured components, effectively smoothing accessible surfaces for bonding or further processing. Nezarati et al. (2025) demonstrated that vibratory finishing significantly improves the surface integrity of AM 316L stainless steel, achieving substantial roughness reduction and enhanced material properties.

In the case study presented further, rotary tumble polishing was applied using coarse and fine media in a staged approach. While larger abrasive particles removed material quickly, they left visible striations. Finer abrasives yielded smoother surfaces, with improved uniformity and tactile quality.

Despite these improvements, mechanical finishing revealed that some regions with limited media contact remained rough, and some areas exhibited potential signs of corrosion. Scanning Electron Microscopy (SEM) showed microstructural discontinuities and possible localized corrosion pits. Moreover, rotary tumbling led to stained surface areas, which may be indicative of early-stage crevice corrosion. These findings underscore the importance of thorough cleaning, including ultrasonic rinsing and passivation after mechanical finishing.

A further concern is the risk of embedding abrasive particles into the surface. SEM imaging showed instances where embedded residues may act as corrosion initiation sites, especially under long-term exposure to the oral environment.

ADDITIONAL SURFACE TREATMENT OPTIONS

While electropolishing and mechanical polishing are the most widely implemented finishing techniques for AM brackets, other advanced or supplementary methods are being explored, such as thermal post-processing where heat treatments like stress-relief annealing and hot isostatic pressing (HIP) reduce internal stresses and porosity, indirectly enhancing surface behavior or laser polishing and surface remelting locally melt a thin surface layer, which re-solidifies into a smoother, more uniform finish. Laser-based methods are particularly valuable for complex or inaccessible geometries but require careful control to avoid thermal distortion.

Additional surface treatment options, such as surface coating of titanium nitride (TiN), hydroxyapatite, or antimicrobial nanolayers, aim to improve wear resistance, reduce ion leaching, and promote biological integration. Coatings are especially relevant in nickel-containing alloys where biocompatibility is a concern.

After discussion of regulatory overview and validation requirements for AM orthodontic brackets in the next chapter, the following chapter will present the case study comparing rotary tumble finishing and electropolishing, which were identified as the most feasible post-processing options for orthodontic brackets. These methods were selected due to their suitability for small medical components, ability to process multiple parts simultaneously, and relative effectiveness in accessing and treating complex geometries – including inner cavities and undercuts – common in custom bracket designs.

REFERENCES

Melia, M. A., Duran, J. G., Koepke, J. R., Saiz, D. J., Jared, B. H., & Schindelholz, E. J. (2020). How build angle and post-processing impact roughness and corrosion of additively manufactured 316L stainless steel. *npj Materials Degradation, 4*, 21. https://doi.org/10.1038/s41529-020-00126-5

Nezarati, M., Sayadi, D., & Hemasian Etefagh, A. (2025). Experimental study on enhancing surface integrity and corrosion resistance in additively manufactured 316L stainless steel through vibratory finishing technique. *Proceedings of the Institution of Mechanical Engineers, Part B: Journal of Engineering Manufacture, 240*, 261–281. https://doi.org/10.1177/09544054241310327

Tyagi, P., Goulet, T., Riso, C., Stephenson, R., Chuenprateep, N., Schlitzer, J., Benton, C., & Garcia-Moreno, F. (2019). Reducing the roughness of internal surface of an additive manufacturing produced 316 steel component by chempolishing and electropolishing. *Additive Manufacturing, 25*, 32–38. https://doi.org/10.1016/j.addma.2018.11.001

Regulatory Framework and Validation Requirements for Additively Manufactured Orthodontic Brackets

5

REGULATION IMPORTANCE FOR ADDITIVELY MANUFACTURED ORTHODONTIC DEVICES

Additive manufacturing (AM) has catalyzed a profound transformation in orthodontic device design and production, enabling a shift from standardized, mass-manufactured components toward highly individualized appliances. Powder-bed fusion (PBF) technologies, particularly selective laser melting (SLM) and direct metal laser sintering (DMLS), allow for the precise fabrication of complex geometries directly from digital models. These systems

DOI: 10.1201/9781003772897-6

provide opportunities to develop orthodontic brackets with customized base curvature, integrated mechanical features, and optimized anatomical conformity, reflecting a broader movement toward personalized digital dentistry (Vafadar et al., 2021).

However, AM introduces material characteristics that differ fundamentally from wrought or machined stainless steel. In AM 316L stainless steel, rapid solidification produces cellular and columnar sub-grain structures, melt-pool boundaries, and non-equilibrium distributions of alloying elements. These features contrast sharply with the equiaxed grain morphology of conventionally processed alloys and influence mechanical performance, fatigue behavior, and corrosion susceptibility (DebRoy et al., 2018; Vukkum & Gupta, 2022). Process-dependent microstructural heterogeneity, combined with the possibility of retained porosity or incomplete melting, creates safety considerations that demand regulatory attention.

The oral environment compounds these concerns. Orthodontic brackets operate in a chemically dynamic and microbiologically rich milieu where fluctuating pH, enzymatic activity, salivary ions, and temperature cycling continuously challenge material stability. Acidic zones produced by dental plaque and biofilms have been shown to accelerate localized corrosion and passive-film breakdown on stainless steel (Eduok & Szpunar, 2020; Xu et al., 2024). Fluoride-containing oral care products, while beneficial to enamel, may destabilize the chromium oxide layer and increase nickel or chromium ion release under certain conditions. These well-documented oral phenomena underscore why bracket materials, especially those with AM-induced microstructural features or surface roughness, must undergo rigorous evaluation prior to clinical use (DelRio et al., 2023).

Given these complexities, regulatory agencies such as the U.S. Food and Drug Administration (FDA) do not evaluate AM brackets as simple variants of existing stainless-steel devices. Instead, the FDA considers AM materials to be process-dependent, meaning their safety and performance characteristics arise from the interplay of powder properties, laser energy input, thermal gradients, and post-processing steps rather than from alloy designation alone. The FDA guidance document on additive manufacturing explicitly highlights the need for detailed process characterization, build parameter control, powder reuse validation, and post-processing standardization, recognizing that even small variations in AM workflow can alter the final device's structure and function (U.S. Food and Drug Administration, 2017).

This regulatory perspective carries significant implications. Manufacturers must demonstrate that their AM workflow, including spanning digital design, powder handling, layer-wise fabrication, heat treatment, surface finishing, and sterilization, consistently produces devices that meet predefined safety, mechanical, and biocompatibility criteria. Compliance requires adherence to global standards such as ISO 13485 (quality management for medical devices), ISO 14971 (risk management), and ISO 10993 (biological evaluation of medical devices). These standards form the backbone of a regulatory strategy that addresses final device performance, the reproducibility, and traceability of the entire manufacturing process.

Structured regulatory evaluation also ensures that the unique risks of AM are addressed before devices reach patients. For instance, as-printed AM surfaces exhibit higher roughness and may retain partially fused particles, increasing frictional forces at the bracket-archwire interface and promoting plaque retention – factors that influence both biomechanics and oral health.

Microstructural heterogeneity may increase susceptibility to pitting or crevice corrosion, particularly in regions with incomplete melting or high surface area. Dimensional drift during electropolishing or thermal processing may alter slot geometry or torque expression. These considerations illustrate why AM brackets must undergo direct mechanical, electrochemical, and biological testing rather than relying on legacy data for traditional stainless-steel materials.

The broader purpose of regulatory oversight is not to constrain innovation but to ensure that the advantages of AM are realized without compromising patient safety. As orthodontics embraces digital workflows, customized geometries, and on-demand manufacturing, a robust regulatory framework provides the foundation for safe implementation. For engineers, this framework highlights the importance of process control and validation. For clinicians, it ensures that AM devices meet the same reliability standards as traditional appliances. For regulatory specialists, it defines the evidence required to evaluate devices produced through non-traditional manufacturing routes.

FDA REGULATORY OVERVIEW FOR ADDITIVELY MANUFACTURED ORTHODONTIC BRACKETS

The FDA regulates orthodontic brackets as Class II medical devices cleared through the 510(k) pathway, where manufacturers must demonstrate substantial equivalence to a predicate device. For conventionally manufactured stainless-steel brackets, this process is straightforward. However, additive manufacturing (AM) introduces microstructural, surface, and geometric differences that require the FDA to evaluate not only the alloy but the entire AM process, from powder sourcing to post-processing.

Under laser powder-bed fusion, stainless steel develops process-dependent features such as columnar grains, melt-pool boundaries, anisotropic properties, and potential porosity. Because such characteristics affect fatigue strength, corrosion behavior, and ion release, the FDA treats AM brackets as technologically distinct from wrought or machined stainless steel. As outlined in the FDA's 2017 AM guidance, manufacturers must provide detailed documentation of powder composition and cleanliness, process parameter controls, environmental conditions during printing, and consistency across builds.

The FDA places significant emphasis on post-processing, since finishing strongly influences surface roughness, passive-film stability, and dimensional precision. Brackets require tight tolerances, and electropolishing or heat treatments can subtly alter slot geometry or tie-wing integrity. Therefore, the FDA expects evidence that finishing produces repeatable mechanical and electrochemical performance.

For device-level evaluation, manufacturers must show that AM brackets meet clinical performance standards for slot accuracy, torque expression, tie-wing strength, friction, and bonding behavior. Additional testing may be required to address AM-specific risks such as porosity-related fracture susceptibility or orientation-dependent strength.

The FDA also requires microstructural and defect characterization through techniques such as microCT, SEM, or optical microscopy to confirm internal consistency and absence of critical defects. Because surface chemistry and oxide stability differ from conventional materials, biocompatibility testing under ISO 10993 must be performed on the final polished device, including cytotoxicity, sensitization, irritation, and chemical characterization.

Together, these expectations reflect the FDA's process-focused approach: AM brackets must demonstrate that all steps of manufacturing, such as powder handling, printing, heat treatment, and finishing, produce devices that match the safety and performance of predicate brackets. This comprehensive evaluation ensures that AM orthodontic devices are clinically reliable despite the unique characteristics introduced by additive manufacturing.

Substantial Equivalence and Predicate Device Challenges in AM Orthodontics

Substantial equivalence (SE) is the foundational requirement for 510(k) clearance. A device must demonstrate the same intended use and comparable technological characteristics to a legally marketed predicate, or show that any differences do not raise new safety or effectiveness concerns. For traditional stainless-steel orthodontic brackets, SE is straightforward because manufacturing methods, material behavior, and performance characteristics are well established. In contrast, additively manufactured brackets introduce new technological characteristics, even when fabricated from the same nominal alloy (316L), that must be explicitly addressed in an SE rationale.

The core regulatory challenge is that AM does not simply replicate the microstructure of wrought or machined stainless steel. Instead, laser powder-bed fusion (LPBF) creates process-dependent microstructures, including cellular and columnar grains, melt-pool boundaries, and varying porosity, that differ significantly from conventional materials (DebRoy et al., 2018; Vukkum & Gupta, 2022). These microstructural differences can affect key performance aspects of orthodontic brackets, such as fatigue strength, tie-wing fracture resistance, torque expression stability, and corrosion behavior. As a result, the FDA views AM brackets as having different technological characteristics, requiring a more robust comparison to the chosen predicate.

Several AM-specific factors influence SE determinations:

- **Microstructure and anisotropy**
  LPBF produces directional solidification patterns and anisotropic properties that are absent in wrought materials. If build orientation influences mechanical performance (e.g., tie-wing strength or slot deformation under load), this must be supported by testing.
- **Porosity and internal defects**
  Traditional brackets exhibit negligible internal porosity. AM brackets may contain lack-of-fusion voids or keyhole pores, depending on energy density. Because porosity affects fracture resistance and fatigue behavior, manufacturers must quantify porosity and demonstrate its clinical insignificance.
- **Surface roughness and oxide chemistry**
  As-printed surfaces retain unmelted particles and stair-step features that increase roughness and may alter corrosion dynamics. Electropolishing mitigates these effects, but also changes geometry. FDA expects before/after measurements to confirm that finishing does not compromise slot tolerances.
- **Corrosion susceptibility and ion release**
  AM stainless steel may show altered passive-film behavior due to microstructural or surface differences (DelRio et al., 2023). Corrosion and nickel/chromium ion release testing must therefore demonstrate equivalence to the predicate.
- **Residual stress and distortion**
  Thermal gradients during AM generate internal stresses that can distort small features. FDA expects validation of stress-relief procedures and evidence of dimensional stability.

Because of these differences, SE for AM brackets must be data-driven rather than assumption-based. Manufacturers typically support SE with bench testing in the following areas:

- Dimensional accuracy and slot tolerance (multiple measurement points).
- Mechanical performance, including tie-wing strength, torque expression, and frictional behavior.
- Corrosion and electrochemical testing under clinically relevant conditions (acidic pH, fluoride exposure).
- Biocompatibility, addressing any AM-related surface effects on cytotoxicity or sensitization (ISO 10993: 2018).
- Surface characterization, including roughness, SEM, and microCT assessment of internal defects.

Additionally, finishing processes (e.g., tumbling, electropolishing, or passivation) must be validated because they can impact geometry and performance.

Most manufacturers select a conventional 316L stainless-steel bracket as the predicate. This is generally acceptable if the AM bracket does not introduce new modes of action or novel design features. However, AM brackets with customized geometry, integrated hooks, or non-traditional mechanical configurations may require expanded justification to show SE for critical performance metrics such as torque expression, bonding behavior, and fracture resistance.

In rare cases, if technological differences are too significant, a De Novo pathway may be required.[1] However, for most AM brackets designed to mimic traditional appliances, SE is achievable with comprehensive mechanical, corrosion, and biocompatibility data.

Substantial equivalence for AM orthodontic brackets requires clear, evidence-based demonstration that AM-related differences, such as microstructure, porosity, surface condition, and dimensional variability, do not introduce new safety or effectiveness concerns. When supported by rigorous bench testing and microstructural characterization, SE is attainable, but it requires more analytical depth than for conventionally manufactured brackets.

---

[1] The FDA De Novo pathway is a special regulatory route for novel, low-to-moderate-risk medical devices that have no existing "predicate" device (a similar, already-marketed device) to compare against for 510(k) clearance, allowing them to become Class I or II devices by establishing new classifications and controls.

Additive Manufacturing-Specific Risks

Additive manufacturing introduces material and process-related risks that differ from conventional metal fabrication and must be addressed explicitly in a 510(k) submission. The FDA views these differences as technological changes that may affect mechanical integrity, corrosion resistance, and biocompatibility.

The key AM-specific risks include:

- **Microstructural variability**
  Rapid solidification creates columnar grains, melt-pool boundaries, and anisotropy that can influence bracket strength and fatigue behavior.
- **Internal porosity and defects**
  Gas pores or lack-of-fusion voids may reduce fracture resistance and must be quantified (e.g., via microCT).
- **Surface roughness and particle adhesion**
  As-printed surfaces retain unmelted particles and stair-step artifacts, increasing friction, plaque retention, and corrosion susceptibility.
- **Passive-film instability and corrosion behavior**
  AM surfaces may exhibit different oxide chemistry, requiring corrosion and ion-release testing under simulated oral conditions.
- **Residual stresses**
  Thermal gradients can distort small features or alter slot geometry; therefore, heat treatment validation is required.
- **Powder handling and contamination risks**
  Variability in powder chemistry, moisture, or oxygen levels can affect melt-pool formation and device consistency.
- **Post-processing sensitivity**
  Finishing steps such as tumbling, electropolishing, or passivation influence both geometry and corrosion performance and must be validated.

The FDA expects manufacturers to identify and mitigate these risks through process validation, dimensional and mechanical testing, corrosion/biocompatibility evaluation, and microstructural characterization. The central regulatory requirement is demonstrating that AM-related differences do not introduce new safety or effectiveness concerns relative to the predicate device.

Predicate Strategy and Regulatory Pathway Considerations

For additively manufactured (AM) orthodontic brackets, the most important element of a successful 510(k) submission is selecting an appropriate predicate and demonstrating that AM-related differences do not introduce new risks. While AM brackets may use the same base alloy (316L stainless steel) as traditional devices, the manufacturing pathway produces meaningful differences, such as microstructure, porosity, roughness, and residual stress, that the FDA considers technological distinctions requiring justification. Therefore, substantial equivalence cannot rely solely on material similarity; it must be supported by evidence that the finished AM bracket performs equivalently to the predicate bracket in clinically relevant ways.

The predicate is typically a conventionally manufactured stainless-steel bracket with similar intended use, prescription, slot dimensions, and bonding interface. The FDA generally accepts this alignment, but AM introduces structural and surface conditions that must be evaluated through testing. These include differences in solidification patterns, internal defects, and surface morphology, all of which may influence fatigue strength, corrosion behavior, ion release, slot accuracy, or tie-wing integrity. As a result, the performance data package becomes central to the predicate argument.

To demonstrate substantial equivalence, manufacturers provide mechanical testing (tie-wing fracture strength, friction, torque expression), dimensional verification before and after finishing, and corrosion/ion release testing under oral conditions. Biocompatibility evaluation is also required, even when the alloy is well established, because AM may alter passive-film chemistry or surface particle retention. To ensure the bracket meets the functional specifications, dimensional changes resulting from material-removing processes like electropolishing must be quantified.

If the AM bracket incorporates patient-specific geometry or integrated features, the FDA focuses on whether these design differences change biomechanical behavior or introduce new safety questions. In most cases, expanded mechanical data and risk analysis can still support substantial equivalence. Only in rare situations, such as devices with fundamentally novel functions, would the FDA consider a De Novo pathway, but this is unlikely for stainless-steel orthodontic brackets.

In summary, predicate selection for AM brackets is achievable but depends on a concise, data-driven demonstration that AM-induced differences do not affect safety or effectiveness. The FDA's review emphasizes validated manufacturing controls and performance metrics, ensuring the AM device behaves like its predicate in clinical use.

BIOCOMPATIBILITY REQUIREMENTS (ISO 10993)

The FDA requires that orthodontic brackets, including AM stainless-steel brackets, undergo biocompatibility evaluation according to the ISO 10993 framework. Even though 316L stainless steel has a long history of safe intraoral use, AM alters key factors such as surface chemistry, passive-film integrity, residual particles, and oxide composition that may affect biological interactions. Therefore, biocompatibility must be demonstrated for the final post-processed device, and not assumed from material designation alone.

The ISO 10993 test battery for a device that contacts oral mucosa for prolonged periods typically includes cytotoxicity, sensitization, irritation, and chemical characterization. For AM brackets, chemical characterization becomes especially important because LPBF processing can modify alloy distribution at the surface and increase the presence of unmelted or partially melted particles, which may influence nickel and chromium ion release. Studies show that oral biofilms, acidic pH, and fluoride compounds can accelerate corrosion and ion leaching from stainless steel, reinforcing the need for robust chemical and corrosion testing (Eduok & Szpunar, 2020; Xu et al., 2024). Thus, the FDA requires manufacturers to show that the final polished bracket meets biological safety criteria.

A central regulatory expectation is that biocompatibility evaluation be integrated with broader process validation. Because AM introduces variability in powder quality, build parameters, and heat treatment, manufacturers must demonstrate consistent biological behavior across production lots. ISO 14971 risk management is used to link biocompatibility hazards, such as ion release, surface residues, and powder contamination, to specific process controls.

In summary, compliance with ISO 10993 for AM orthodontic brackets requires a process-aware strategy: chemical and biological testing must reflect how AM fabrication and finishing influence the final device's interactions with oral tissues. The FDA expects manufacturers to provide a scientifically justified, test-supported demonstration that the finished bracket is safe for long-term intraoral use.

MANUFACTURING AND FINISHING PROCESS VALIDATION FOR AM ORTHODONTIC BRACKETS

Ensuring consistent quality in AM orthodontic brackets requires validation of both the manufacturing workflow and the finishing processes that finalize the device. The FDA evaluates AM brackets based on both performance testing and the reliability of the entire manufacturing process, from powder handling to final surface finishing, to ensure consistency with tested samples. This approach is grounded in ISO 13485 quality management principles and the IQ/OQ/PQ validation framework.

Manufacturing Workflow Validation (IQ/OQ/PQ)

Manufacturing workflow validation for AM orthodontic brackets is typically structured according to the Installation Qualification (IQ), Operational Qualification (OQ), and Performance Qualification (PQ) framework, as defined in FDA process validation guidance and supported by ISO 13485 requirements for medical device manufacturing (FDA, 2011; ISO 13485:2016).

Installation Qualification (IQ) establishes that AM equipment and supporting systems, including laser powder-bed fusion machines, inert-gas supply systems, powder sieves, recoaters, and post-processing tools, are installed, calibrated, and configured in accordance with manufacturer specifications and validated procedures. Environmental controls such as oxygen concentration, humidity, and temperature are verified during IQ because deviations in these parameters can directly influence melt-pool stability, porosity formation, microstructure, and surface quality in AM stainless-steel components.

Operational Qualification (OQ) confirms that critical process parameters such as laser power, scan speed, hatch spacing, layer thickness, build atmosphere purity, and powder handling conditions operate within predefined and validated ranges. Because the microstructure, density, and surface condition of AM parts are inherently process-dependent, OQ ensures that expected variations in these parameters do not result in unacceptable changes to bracket geometry, internal integrity, or surface characteristics (FDA, 2011; ISO 13485: 2016).

Performance Qualification (PQ) demonstrates that the fully validated manufacturing workflow consistently produces orthodontic brackets that meet predefined specifications under routine production conditions. PQ typically includes microstructural verification, dimensional inspection of critical features (particularly slot dimensions), mechanical testing (e.g., tie-wing strength and deformation), and surface or corrosion performance metrics. Demonstration of lot-to-lot reproducibility is central to PQ, as regulatory authorities require evidence that the device evaluated in a 510(k) submission accurately represents ongoing commercial production capability (FDA, 2011).

Finishing Process Validation and Regulatory Importance

For orthodontic brackets, finishing processes are essential because, as discussed above, as-printed surfaces exhibit elevated roughness, partially fused powder, and micro-defects that can affect friction, plaque accumulation, bond strength, and corrosion behavior. The FDA therefore expects manufacturers to validate each finishing step and quantify its effect on device safety and performance (FDA, 2017).

To validate metrics, the FDA expects manufacturers to provide:

- Before and after roughness measurements.
- Before and after dimensional analysis.
- Demonstration of improved corrosion resistance.
- Evidence of repeatability across multiple builds.
- Confirmation that finishing does not introduce new defects such as microcracks or distortion.

The electropolishing case study presented in the next chapter supports this regulatory requirement. By demonstrating substantial reductions in surface roughness, improved corrosion resistance, minimal geometric distortion, and a clinically acceptable final surface, the work provides empirical evidence for finishing process validation in AM orthodontic brackets.

REFERENCES

DebRoy, T., Wei, H. L., Zuback, J. S., Mukherjee, T., Elmer, J. W., Milewski, J. O., Beese, A. M., Wilson-Heid, A., De, A., & Zhang, W. (2018). Additive manufacturing of metallic components: Process, structure and properties.

Progress in Materials Science, 92, 112–224. https://doi.org/10.1016/j.pmatsci.2017.10.001

DelRio, F. W., Khan, R. M., Heiden, M. J., Melia, M. A., Rodelas, J. M., & Schindelholz, E. J. (2023). Porosity, roughness, and passive film morphology influence the corrosion behavior of 316L stainless steel manufactured by laser powder bed fusion. *Journal of Manufacturing Processes, 103*, 654–662. https://doi.org/10.1016/j.jmapro.2023.07.062

Eduok, U., & Szpunar, J. A. (2020). In vitro corrosion studies of stainless-steel dental substrates during *Porphyromonas gingivalis* biofilm growth in artificial saliva solutions. *RSC Advances, 10*(52), 31280–31294. https://doi.org/10.1039/D0RA05500J

International Organization for Standardization. (2016). *ISO 13485:2016 – Medical devices – Quality management systems – Requirements for regulatory purposes.* ISO.

International Organization for Standardization. (2018). *ISO 10993-1:2018 – Biological evaluation of medical devices – Part 1: Evaluation and testing within a risk management process.* ISO.

International Organization for Standardization. (2019). *ISO 14971:2019 – Medical devices – Application of risk management to medical devices.* ISO.

U.S. Food and Drug Administration. (2011). *Process validation: General principles and practices.* U.S. Department of Health and Human Services. Retrieved from www.fda.gov/files/drugs/published/Process-Validation--General-Principles-and-Practices.pdf?utm_source=chatgpt.com

U.S. Food and Drug Administration. (2017). *Technical considerations for additive manufactured medical devices: Guidance for industry and Food and Drug Administration staff.* Retrieved from www.fda.gov/media/97633/download

Vafadar, A., Guzzomi, F., Rassau, A., & Hayward, K. (2021). Advances in metal additive manufacturing: A review of common processes, industrial applications, and current challenges. *Applied Sciences, 11*(3), 1213. https://doi.org/10.3390/app11031213

Vukkum, V. B., & Gupta, R. K. (2022). Review on corrosion performance of laser powder-bed fusion printed 316L stainless steel: Effect of processing parameters, manufacturing defects, post-processing, feedstock, and microstructure. *Materials & Design, 221*, 110874. https://doi.org/10.1016/j.matdes.2022.110874

Xu, W., Yu, F., Addison, O., Davenport, A. J., & Liu, Y. (2024). Microbial corrosion of metallic biomaterials in the oral environment. *Acta Biomaterialia, 184*, 22–36. https://doi.org/10.1016/j.actbio.2024.06.032

Case Study

Surface Characterization Techniques and Baseline Analysis

6

STUDY HYPOTHESES

Based on findings from the literature and clinical requirements for high-performance biocompatible brackets, this study investigates two key hypotheses:

1. **Rotary tumble finishing** with appropriate abrasive media can produce a smooth surface topography on additively manufactured (AM) stainless steel brackets without compromising surface chemistry.
2. **Electropolishing** can reduce surface roughness and enhance intrinsic corrosion resistance.

In both cases, the surface quality of traditionally manufactured brackets serves as the performance benchmark.

To rigorously evaluate the proposed hypotheses, an integrated surface characterization protocol encompassing both qualitative and quantitative analyses was implemented. Quantitative surface roughness parameters were measured using a Hirox KH-7700 digital microscope, which employs focal stacking to generate high-resolution, three-dimensional reconstructions with extended depth of field. Complementary chemical and elemental surface composition assessments were conducted via X-ray Photoelectron Spectroscopy

DOI: 10.1201/9781003772897-7

(XPS) and Energy-Dispersive X-ray Spectroscopy (EDS), ensuring a comprehensive evaluation of both topographical and compositional attributes. Detailed methodologies and corresponding analytical outcomes for each technique are presented in the subsequent sections.

SURFACE CHARACTERIZATION BY HIROX KH-7700 DIGITAL MICROSCOPE

Surface roughness was evaluated as a key performance parameter of the brackets using a Hirox KH-7700 digital microscope. After selecting the measurement regions, data collection and analysis were conducted along longitudinal (Y-axis) and transverse (X-axis) directions within each region (Figure 6.1a, b). The corresponding surface profiles, illustrating vertical deviations and centerlines, are presented in Figure 6.1(c) and (d) for the 3D-printed bracket.

Microscopic images were analyzed to calculate the arithmetic average surface roughness (Ra) for each region. The Ra value represents the average of absolute vertical deviations from the mean surface line and is defined by the following equation:

$$R_a = \sum_{i=1}^{n} \frac{|y_i|}{n}, \tag{6.1}$$

where y_i – is the absolute vertical deviation from the centerline, and n is the number of measurement points within the analyzed area (ISO 4287:1997/ 2021).

SURFACE CHARACTERIZATION BY X-RAY PHOTOELECTRON SPECTROSCOPY (XPS)

XPS, a highly surface-sensitive technique, was used to detect elemental composition and chemical states within the top few nanometers of the bracket surface. The system includes various excitation sources (Mg Kα, Al Kα, and monochromatic X-rays), and spectral processing was conducted using CasaXPS software.

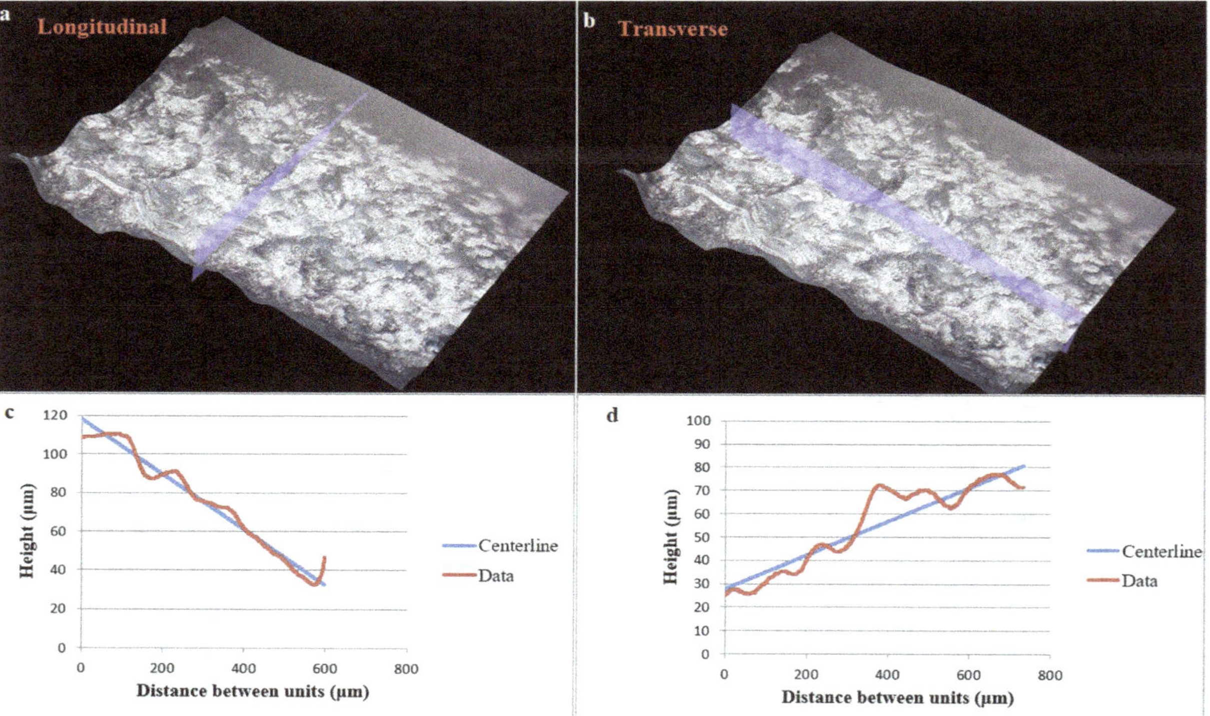

FIGURE 6.1 Directions for measurements. An example of the archwire area of the 3D-printed bracket: (a) longitudinal direction, (b) transverse direction, (c) surface profile derived from longitudinal measurements, (d) surface profile derived from transverse measurements.

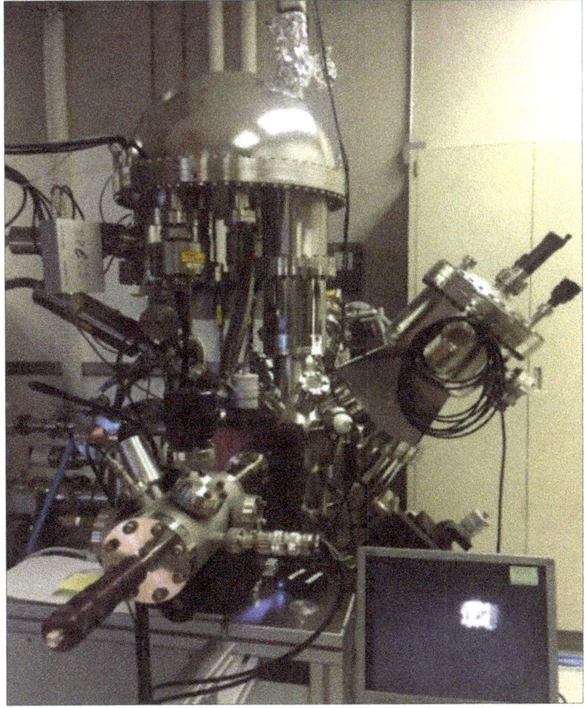

FIGURE 6.2   X-ray Photoelectron Spectroscopy Apparatus.

Figure 6.2 presents the XPS machine, and Figure 6.3 illustrates the working principle of XPS: only photoelectrons emitted from the topmost atomic layers escape with enough kinetic energy to generate meaningful spectra, while deeper electrons lose energy through scattering.

The kinetic energy (KE) of photoelectrons emitted from a material's surface during XPS analysis is governed by the equation:

$$KE = hv - BE - \phi_s.$$

(6.2)

where:

- hv is the photon energy of the incident X-ray,
- BE is the binding energy of the electron within the atom,
- ϕ_s is the work function of the spectrometer.

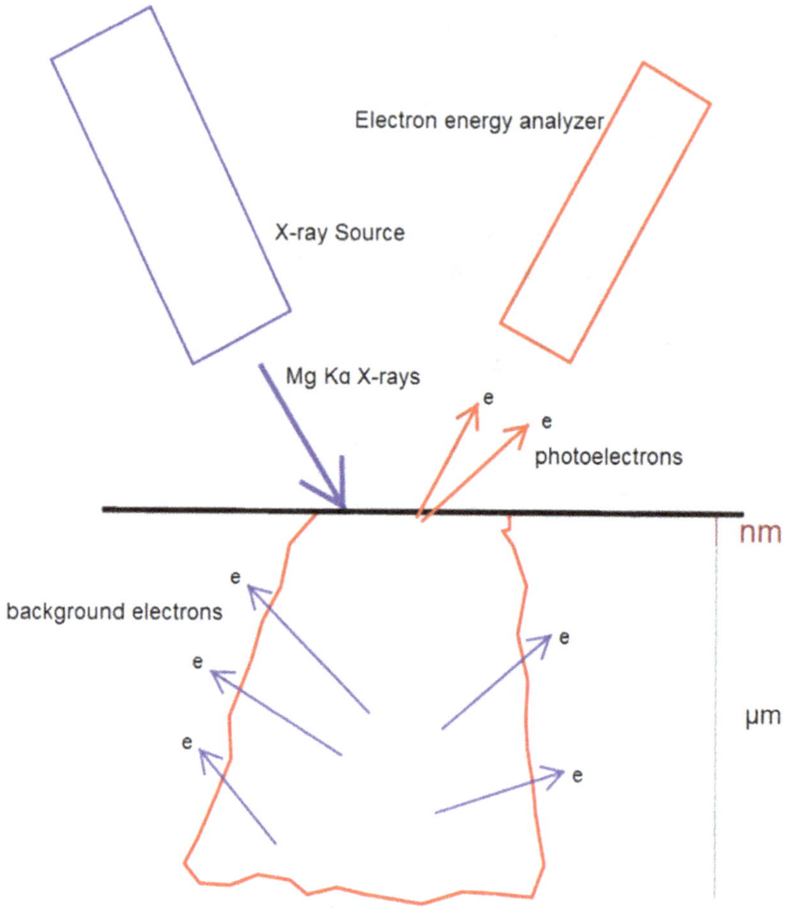

FIGURE 6.3   XPS operating principle.

This relationship is well established and forms the basis of quantitative XPS analysis (Watts & Wolstenholme, 2020). The equation allows for the calculation of binding energies, which are characteristic of specific elements and their chemical states.

In this study, CasaXPS software was used to process the acquired XPS spectra. The software calculates binding energy values by determining the energy difference between the initial and final quantum states of the emitted photoelectrons. Accurate energy referencing and spectral fitting were used to assess the surface chemistry of 3D printed brackets before and after surface finishing treatments.

ENERGY-DISPERSIVE X-RAY SPECTROSCOPY (EDS)

EDS is a complementary technique to XPS, used to determine the elemental composition of materials. Unlike XPS, which is highly surface-sensitive, EDS analyzes the bulk composition – penetrating several micrometers below the surface. In this study, EDS was performed using a Scanning Electron Microscope (SEM) equipped with an EDS detector (Figure 6.4).

Each chemical element exhibits a characteristic emission spectrum, producing a unique set of peaks corresponding to electron transitions between inner and outer shells (Goldstein et al., 2003). When the sample is exposed to a high-energy electron beam, inner-shell electrons are ejected, and the resulting electron vacancies are filled by higher-energy electrons. This transition releases element-specific X-rays, which are captured and analyzed to determine the elemental profile. This technique was essential for verifying the material composition of 3D printed bracket samples and identifying localized chemical inhomogeneities.

Thus, it was hypothesized that the rotary tumble finishing process would improve surface topography by reducing surface roughness, while electropolishing would enhance both surface smoothness and chemical composition – particularly by increasing the surface chromium content. These improvements aimed to replicate or surpass the surface quality observed in conventionally manufactured orthodontic brackets.

Collectively, the integration of high-resolution surface topography analysis (Hirox KH-7700), surface chemical characterization (XPS), and bulk compositional assessment (SEM/EDS) enabled a comprehensive evaluation of both morphological and chemical parameters central to the proposed hypotheses. This multi-modal approach ensured that topographical variations, elemental distributions, and subsurface compositional uniformity were thoroughly assessed, thereby providing a robust basis for hypothesis validation.

CHARACTERIZATION OF TRADITIONAL AND ORIGINAL AM BRACKETS

The conventional bracket exhibited a consistently smooth and reflective surface across the inspected regions. For surface roughness measurements, two specific areas were selected: the upper portion of the bracket and the archwire

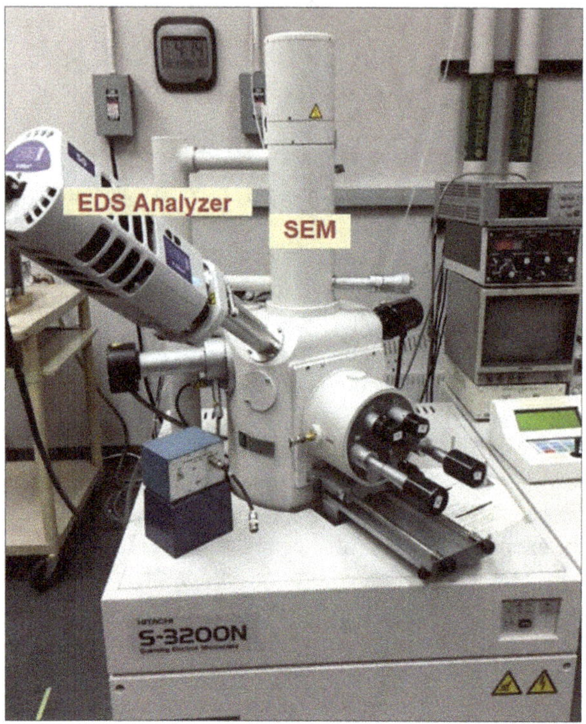

FIGURE 6.4   Energy-Dispersive X-ray Spectroscopy Apparatus.

slot region. Figure 6.5 demonstrates: (a) the traditionally machined bracket in 50× magnification, (b) AM bracket in 50× magnification, (c) archwire region and (e) upper portion of the traditionally machined bracket, and (d) archwire region, and (f) upper portion of the AM bracket in 350× magnification. Surface morphology analysis indicated that the AM bracket possessed markedly higher roughness compared to the conventional bracket.

Longitudinal (Y-axis) and transverse (X-axis) measurement directions were selected for both the archwire slot and the upper bracket areas, as was presented in Figure 6.1.

The initial arithmetic average surface roughness values for the conventional and AM brackets are summarized in Table 6.1.

The overall average surface roughness (Ra) for each bracket was calculated by averaging the values obtained from the selected areas, as shown below:

$$Average\ R_a = \frac{1}{4}\left(R_{a\,X\,archwire} + R_{a\,Y\,archwire} + R_{a\,X\,upper} + R_{a\,Y\,upper}\right) \quad (6.3)$$

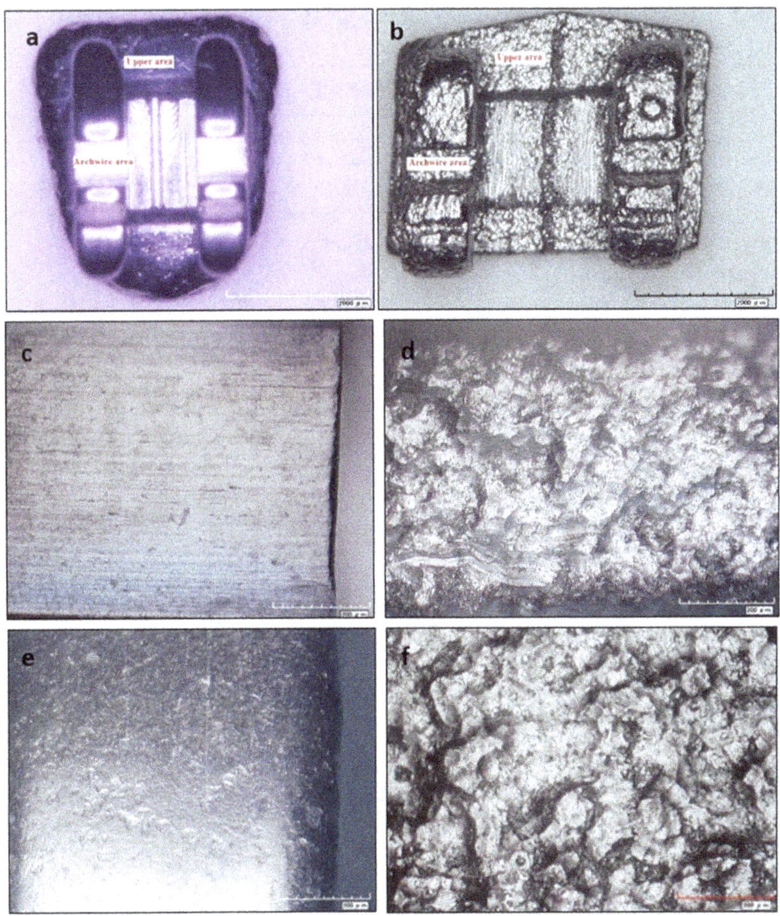

FIGURE 6.5 Hirox microscope images of conventional and additively manufactured (AM) brackets: (a,b) overall views at 50×; (c,d) archwire regions at 350×; (e,f) upper regions at 350×.

Based on the results in Table 6.1, the average Ra of the conventional bracket was 2.02 μm, whereas the 3D-printed bracket exhibited an average Ra of 4.19 μm, approximately twice that of the conventionally machined counterpart.

The arithmetic average surface roughness of the traditional bracket served as a reference value for the investigated surface roughness of the additively manufactured parts to determine the effectiveness of the applied methods.

The surface characterization methods established in this chapter provide the analytical foundation for the experimental investigations that follow. By defining baseline surface roughness, morphology, and chemical composition

TABLE 6.1 Arithmetic average surface roughness (Ra) of as-manufactured brackets

MEASURED PART	SURFACE ROUGHNESS R_A (μm)				
	ARCHWIRE AREA		UPPER AREA		
	ALONG X	ALONG Y	ALONG X	ALONG Y	AVERAGE R_A
Conventional bracket	1.19	2.42	2.17	2.3	2.02
AM bracket	4.84	3.17	5.64	3.14	4.19

for both conventionally manufactured and additively manufactured brackets, this framework enables objective assessment of post-processing effects. The subsequent chapters apply these techniques to evaluate two candidate finishing strategies examining their influence on surface topography, chemistry, dimensional stability, and corrosion-related indicators. Through systematic application of the characterization protocol presented here, the case study chapters quantify how each finishing method alters clinically relevant surface properties and determine their suitability for producing biocompatible, high-performance orthodontic brackets.

REFERENCES

Goldstein, J. I., Newbury, D. E., Joy, D. C., Lyman, C. E., Echlin, P., Lifshin, E., Sawyer, L., & Michael, J. R. (2003). *Scanning electron microscopy and X-ray microanalysis* (3rd ed.). Springer. https://doi.org/10.1007/978-1-4615-0215-9

International Organization for Standardization. (1997). *ISO 4287:1997 – Geometrical product specifications (GPS) – Surface texture: Profile method – Terms, definitions and surface texture parameters (reaffirmed 2021)*. ISO.

Watts, J. F., & Wolstenholme, J. (2020). *An introduction to surface analysis by XPS and AES* (2nd ed.). Wiley. ISBN 9781119417467.

Case Study
Rotary Tumble Finishing of Additively Manufactured Orthodontic Brackets

7

PROCESS OVERVIEW

In rotary tumble finishing, the workpiece is placed in a rotating container together with abrasive media. As previously noted, this method is particularly suitable for components with intricate geometries, provided that an appropriate media type is selected. The hardness, particle size, and shape of the abrasive were systematically evaluated to determine the optimal media for stainless steel brackets.

Silicon carbide and aluminum oxide were selected as tumbling media based on their well-documented performance in vibratory finishing of stainless steel components, where ceramic media often incorporates these abrasives for effective grinding and polishing (Sharretts Plating Company, 2023). While no recent peer-reviewed studies explicitly identify alumina or SiC media in tumbling processes for bracket-scale components, their widespread industrial use underscores their suitability for post-processing intricate geometries.

DOI: 10.1201/9781003772897-8

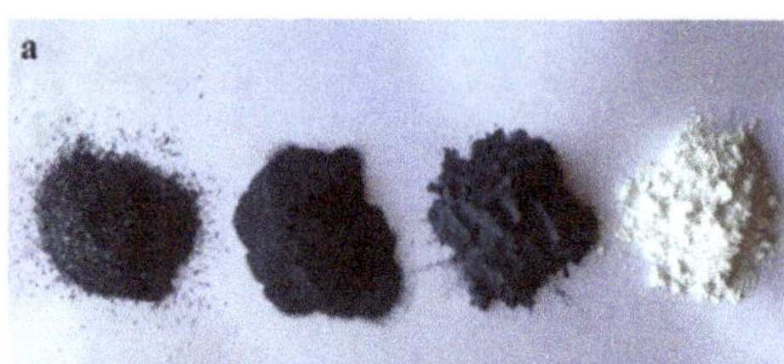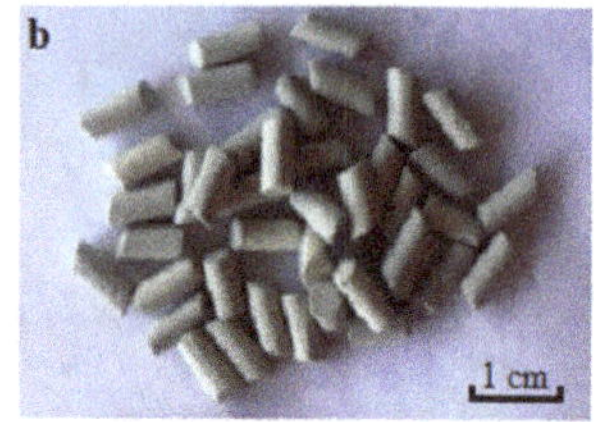

FIGURE 7.1   Abrasive media for mechanical finishing: a) grit F60/90, F150/220, F500, F8000 (from left to right), b) ceramic pellets.

The grit sizes were selected in accordance with FEPA standards (Federation of European Producers of Abrasives, 2006), specifically FEPA-Standard 42-1:2006 for macrogrits (silicon carbide F60/90, F150/220, F500), and FEPA-Standard 42-2:2006 for microgrits (aluminum oxide F8000) (Figure 7.1 a). Ceramic pellets were also added as filler media to enhance grit distribution and improve finishing forces (Figure 7.1b).

Mechanical finishing was performed in a 2-lb rotary barrel containing the abrasive media, the parts, and water, following the procedure detailed below. Grit size and processing time were adjusted after each cycle based on measured surface roughness. The workflow was:

1. Measure the initial surface roughness of the 3D-printed bracket.
2. Conduct rotary tumble finishing with coarse grit (F60/90); adjust duration as needed.
3. Evaluate visible improvements using optical microscopy.
4. Measure the surface roughness of the processed part.
5. Repeat steps 2–4 using finer grits (F150/220, F500, F8000), adjusting time and sequence accordingly.
6. Record surface roughness values after each step.

ROTARY TUMBLE FINISHING: CHARACTERIZATION OF AM BRACKETS

The experiment began with measurement of the initial surface roughness of the as-built 3D-printed sample, followed by application of the abrasive grits as specified in the experimental protocol. Changes in the surface appearance of the archwire slot and the upper bracket area are summarized in Figure 7.2, while the corresponding surface roughness values are presented in Table 7.1.

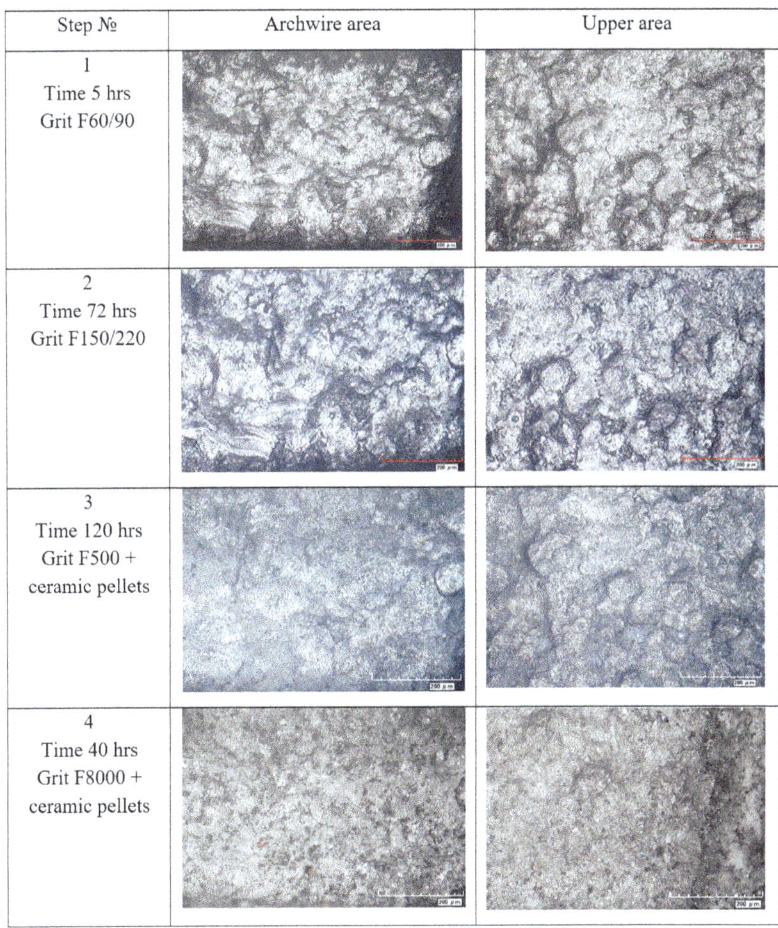

Step №	Archwire area	Upper area
1 Time 5 hrs Grit F60/90		
2 Time 72 hrs Grit F150/220		
3 Time 120 hrs Grit F500 + ceramic pellets		
4 Time 40 hrs Grit F8000 + ceramic pellets		

FIGURE 7.2 Changes of surface appearance of the rotary tumbled AM bracket, as observed by Hirox microscope (350×).

TABLE 7.1 Arithmetic average surface roughness of the finished sample

STEP NO*	TOTAL TIME (HOURS)	GRIT	SURFACE ROUGHNESS R_A (μm)				AVERAGE R_A
			ARCHWIRE AREA		UPPER AREA		
			ALONG X	ALONG Y	ALONG X	ALONG Y	
0	0	0	4.84	3.17	5.64	3.14	4.19
1	5	F60/90	4.51	7.11	4.42	3.32	4.84
2	77	F150/220	4.28	2.93	4.01	3.87	3.77
3	197	F500	3.24	3.09	3.64	3.13	3.28
4	237	F8000	3.43	2.69	2.55	1.60	2.56

DISCUSSION OF SURFACE ROUGHNESS RESULTS

The initial as-built 3D-printed bracket (Figure 6.5d, f, Chapter 6) exhibited a relatively high average surface roughness (Ra) of 4.19 μm, with the archwire slot showing more pronounced irregularities than the upper bracket area. Following the first rotary tumble finishing stage with coarse grit (F60/90), the average Ra increased slightly to 4.84 μm. This temporary increase can be attributed to the aggressive action of the coarse abrasive, which may have removed high asperities but also introduced new surface scratches, particularly evident in the Y-direction of the archwire area (7.11 μm).

Subsequent processing with intermediate grit (F150/220) over a total of 77 h produced a marked improvement, reducing the average Ra to 3.77 μm. This stage effectively mitigated the deeper grooves from the coarse step, resulting in a more uniform surface texture across both measured areas.

Referring to Figure 7.2, after incorporating ceramic pellets, the surface appeared smoother compared to the first-stage images. The pellets facilitated more uniform grit distribution and contributed to force generation within the rotary barrel, thereby enabling more effective material removal and enhanced finishing efficiency. Further refinement with fine grit (F500) brought the average Ra down to 3.28 μm after 197 h of total processing time. At this stage, both the X- and Y-direction measurements showed consistent reductions, indicating effective smoothing of residual micro-scale irregularities.

The final polishing step using very fine aluminum oxide grit (F8000) achieved the lowest average Ra of 2.56 μm. This represents an overall reduction of approximately 39% compared to the as-built surface, with the most significant improvements observed in the upper bracket area (Ra along Y reduced from 3.13 μm to 1.60 μm).

The progression of results confirms the expected trend of gradual surface refinement over time with decreasing abrasive grit size; Figure 7.3 shows the surface roughness trend. However, the initial increase in Ra after coarse grit processing highlights the importance of multi-stage finishing, as coarse media alone may degrade surface quality before subsequent polishing stages restore and enhance smoothness.

These findings support the original hypothesis by demonstrating that a controlled, multi-stage rotary tumble finishing process, optimized with appropriate abrasive grits and aided by ceramic pellets, can substantially improve

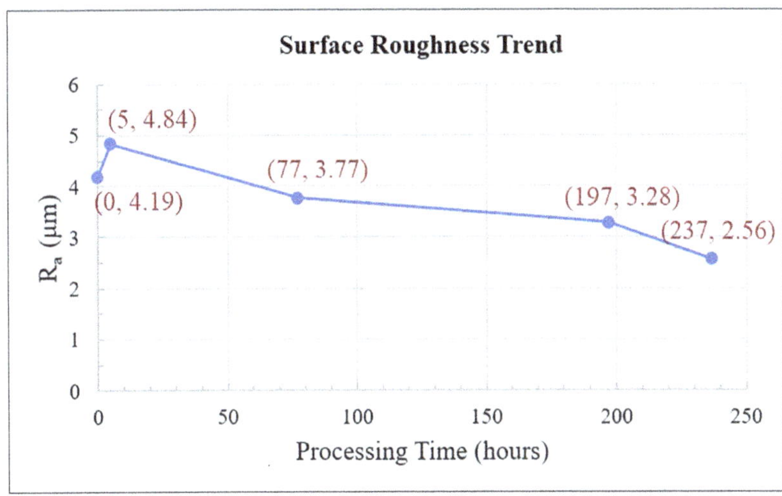

FIGURE 7.3   Variation of surface roughness (Ra) with finishing time.

TABLE 7.2   Dimensional measurements of the initial and finished brackets

DIRECTION	INITIAL DIMENSION (I) (μm)	FINISHED DIMENSION (F) (μm)	DIMENSIONAL CHANGE $\Delta = I - F$ (μm)
Horizontal	4430	4349	81
Vertical	3253	3191	62

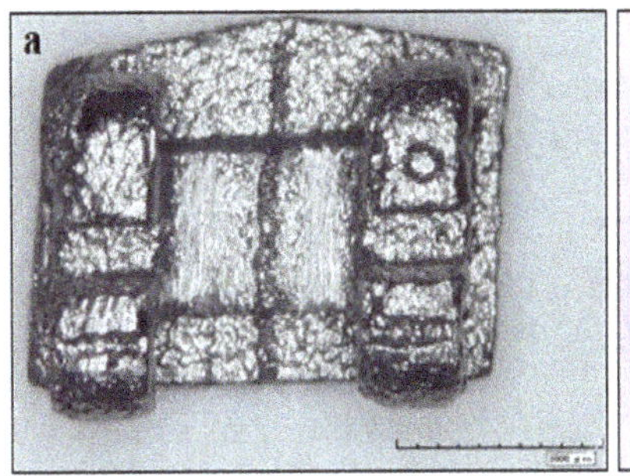
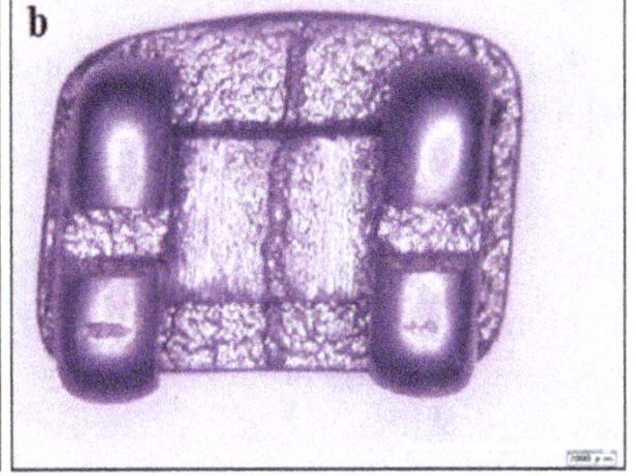

FIGURE 7.4   Hirox microscope images (50x) of the bracket: a) as-built, (b) after rotary tumble finishing.

the surface quality of 3D-printed stainless steel orthodontic brackets. However, the conventional bracket exhibited a lower average roughness of 2.02 μm, indicating that even after mechanical finishing, the 3D-printed part did not fully match the surface smoothness of its conventionally manufactured counterpart.

EFFECT OF MECHANICAL FINISHING ON BRACKET GEOMETRY

As shown in Figure 7.4, rotary tumble finishing altered the bracket's geometry, with edges becoming noticeably rounded due to the rotational action of the process. Dimensional changes were quantified using a digital microscope at 50× magnification (Table 7.2).

Measurements indicated that the process removed approximately 81 μm in the horizontal direction and 62 μm in the vertical direction. These dimensional reductions should be taken into account during bracket design to ensure the desired post-processing geometry.

SURFACE DISCOLORATION AND POTENTIAL CORROSION FOLLOWING ROTARY TUMBLE FINISHING

Further inspection revealed an unexpected finding directly relevant to Hypothesis 1, which proposed that rotary tumble finishing with appropriate abrasive media can produce a smooth surface topography on additively manufactured stainless steel brackets without compromising surface chemistry. Upon completion of the rotary tumble finishing process, several discolored regions were observed on the bracket surface. This prompted a re-evaluation of the process, despite its demonstrated ability to reduce surface roughness. Although conclusive evidence of active corrosion could not be established, possible rusty spots were visible in the archwire area under Hirox microscope magnification (Figure 7.5). These observations suggest that, while rotary tumble finishing was effective in improving surface topography, it may have compromised surface chemistry – potentially through disruption of the passive oxide layer, particularly if the surface contained insufficient free chromium to maintain effective passivation.

Recent studies have significantly advanced our understanding of corrosion in additively manufactured stainless steels. While Laleh et al. (2019) demonstrated that SLM-produced 316L stainless steel exhibits enhanced resistance to classical intergranular corrosion, even after sensitization, this behavior does not preclude susceptibility to other corrosion modes. More recent work by DelVecchio et al. (2024) showed that the metastable cellular microstructures characteristic of LPBF 316L contain Cr- and Mo-depleted regions that act as preferential initiation sites for localized corrosion, highlighting the vulnerability of additively manufactured microstructures to corrosion under clinically relevant conditions.

Even surface microstructure integrity can be compromised by mechanical post-processing, such as rotary tumbling, which may disrupt passive films or introduce residual stress, increasing susceptibility to corrosion. Additionally, elemental segregation and, under certain thermal histories, carbide precipitation can locally deplete chromium, reducing surface passivity and promoting localized corrosion. Such mechanisms have been documented in both laser-based additive manufacturing systems and conventional fabrication routes (e.g., Li et al., 2013; Ko et al., 2021).

Taken together, these findings emphasize that the corrosion behavior of AM stainless steel brackets depends not only on alloy microstructure but also on post-processing. Furthermore, the use of the same additive manufacturing

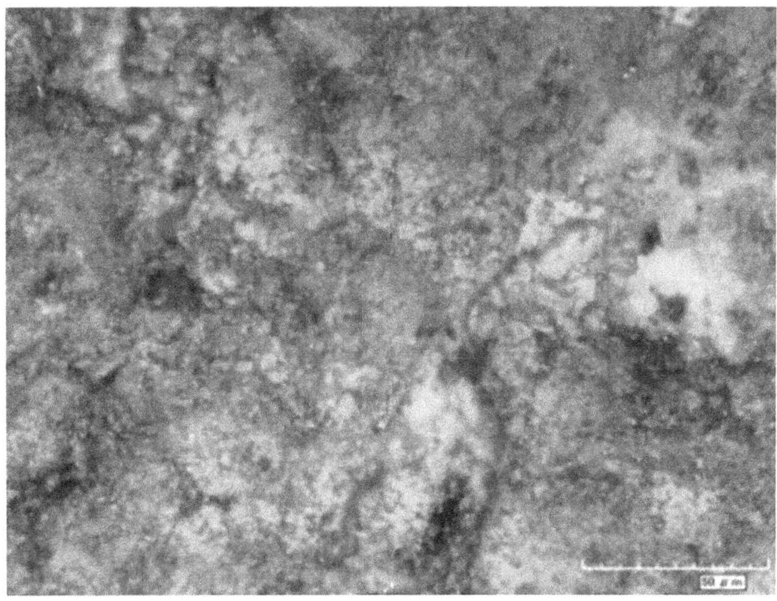

FIGURE 7.5 Hirox microscope image of the archwire area; scale bar = 50 μm.

apparatus for different alloys increases the risk of residual foreign particles adhering to the printed surface; these contaminants can serve as corrosion initiation sites if not removed during post-processing.

These observations reinforce the finding that while rotary tumble finishing can enhance surface smoothness, it may also alter the surface chemistry in a manner that compromises corrosion resistance. Consequently, the selection of post-processing methods for additively manufactured orthodontic brackets must account for both geometric and electrochemical performance requirements.

SURFACE CHARACTERIZATION BY X-RAY PHOTOELECTRON SPECTROSCOPY (XPS)

In addition to surface roughness evaluation using the digital microscope, XPS was employed to determine the elemental and chemical composition of the surfaces of 3D-printed brackets before and after mechanical finishing. Although visibly rusty areas were observed on the top side of the finished bracket, the back side of the bracket was selected for analysis due to limitations in sample positioning within the instrument. Prior to analysis, the samples were cleaned with an alcohol solution and stored in glass containers.

The XPS spectrum of the as-built 3D-printed bracket (Figure 7.6) revealed the surface to be composed primarily of carbon (68.2 at%), oxygen (30.8 at%), and chromium (1.1 at%). As discussed in Chapter 6, XPS probes only the outermost ≈2 nm of the surface; consequently, the measured composition is strongly influenced by surface films, oxides, and adsorbed contaminants. The low metal content likely reflects the irregular topography of the sampled area, which can hinder accurate measurement. Elevated surface carbon is commonly observed in additively manufactured stainless steels and may arise from adventitious contamination and/or carbon-rich surface phases. In AM 316L, such carbon enrichment has been associated with microstructural heterogeneity and localized chromium depletion, which can compromise passivity and promote corrosion susceptibility (Ko et al., 2021). Binding energy analysis further suggests the possible presence of chromium–carbon bonding states, consistent with altered near-surface chromium distribution and reduced chromium availability in the passive film (Boonruang & Sanumang, 2021).

The XPS spectrum of the mechanically finished bracket (Figure 7.7) showed carbon (78.7 at%) and oxygen (21.3 at%) as the dominant elements, with no detectable metallic species. Given the high sensitivity of XPS, residual

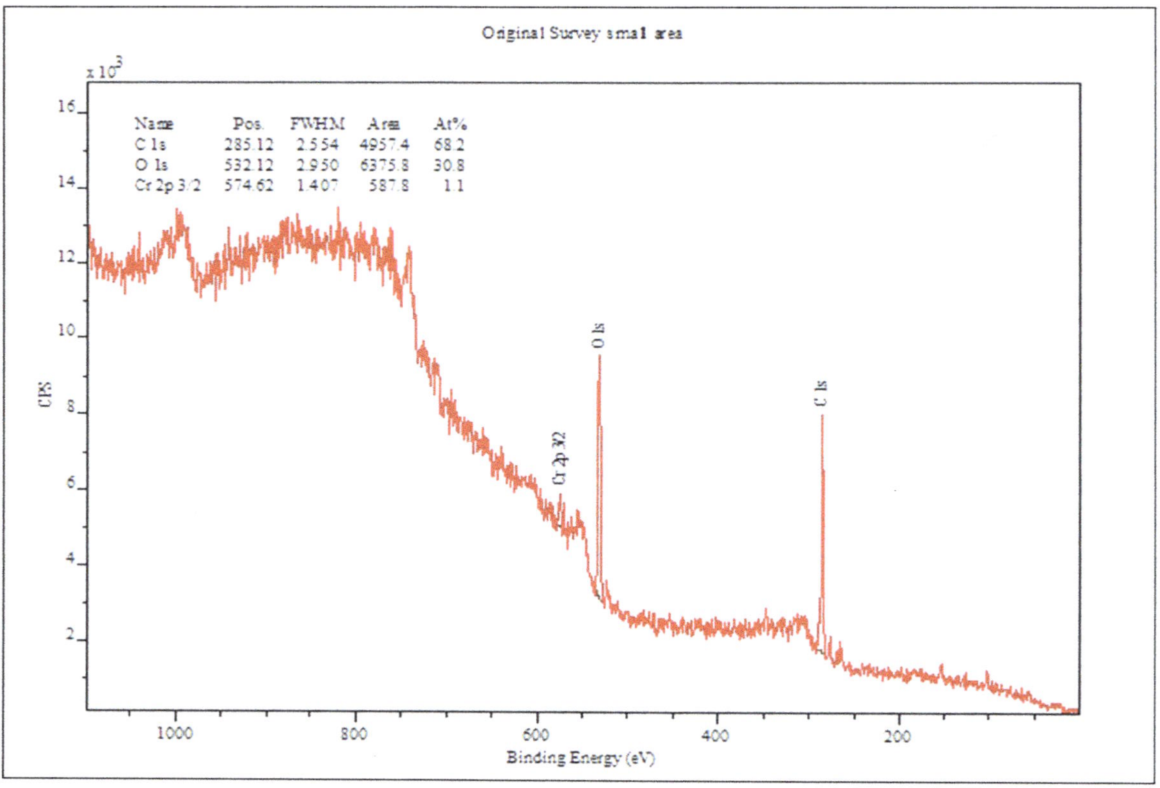

FIGURE 7.6   XPS spectrum of the as-built 3D-printed orthodontic bracket surface.

TABLE 7.3   Surface elemental composition (at%) of as-built and mechanically finished AM stainless steel brackets obtained by XPS

	ELEMENT	AS-BUILT BRACKET (AT%)	MECHANICALLY FINISHED BRACKET (AT%)
1	Carbon (C)	68.2	78.7
2	Oxygen (O)	30.8	21.3
3	Chromium (Cr)	1.1	ND
4	Metals (Others)	ND	ND

contamination could account for the absence of metals. The grooved morphology of the back side of the bracket likely impeded the complete removal of contaminants during cleaning, further influencing the measured composition. The XPS results are also presented in Table 7.3.

These results suggest that rotary tumble finishing, while effective in reducing surface roughness, may under certain conditions disrupt the integrity of the protective oxide layer or alter near-surface chemistry, potentially increasing susceptibility to localized corrosion. While smoother AM 316L surfaces are generally associated with higher breakdown potentials and improved corrosion resistance (Melia et al., 2020), this benefit is contingent on preservation of surface chemistry and passive film stability. Using in situ liquid-cell transmission electron microscopy (TEM), Tian et al. (2022) observed that corrosion initiation in LPBF 316L preferentially occurs along dislocation-cell (cellular substructure) boundaries, indicating that AM-specific microstructural features can act as early sites for localized attack. More recently, Sangoi et al. (2025) showed that pitting susceptibility and repassivation behavior in LPBF 316L are anisotropic and depend on build orientation and thermal history, suggesting that both manufacturing and post-processing must be optimized for corrosion performance.

From a post-processing perspective, Prochaska and Hildreth (2022) demonstrated that chemically accelerated vibratory finishing (CAVF) can mitigate corrosion-related vulnerabilities in stainless steels by removing mechanically and chemically unstable near-surface layers associated with carbide formation and chromium depletion, resulting in improved breakdown potentials. Together, these studies confirm that the choice of post-processing strategy is critical for geometric refinement as well as for preserving or enhancing the electrochemical stability of AM stainless steels.

Consequently, when applying rotary tumble finishing to orthodontic brackets, process parameters should be selected with consideration for both mechanical and electrochemical outcomes, potentially in combination with complementary treatments that restore or improve passivation.

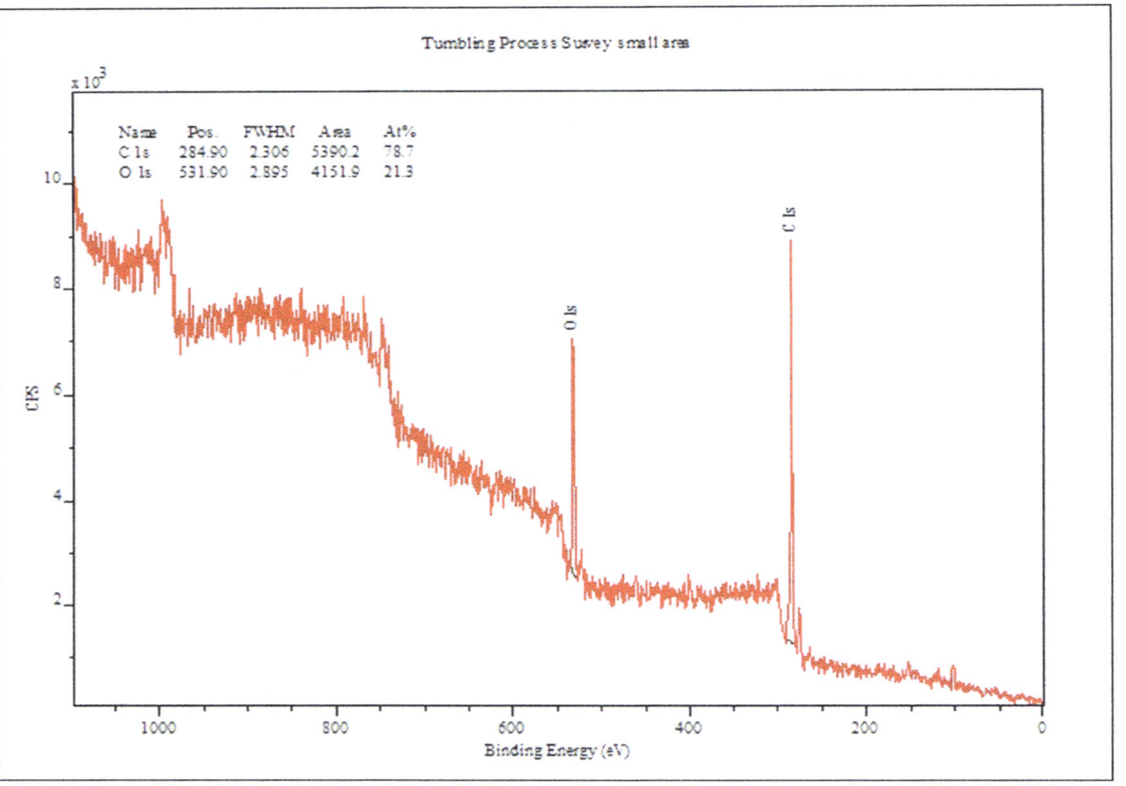

FIGURE 7.7 XPS spectrum of the mechanically finished 3D-printed bracket surface.

SURFACE CHARACTERIZATION BY ENERGY-DISPERSIVE X-RAY SPECTROSCOPY (EDS)

Energy-Dispersive X-ray Spectroscopy (EDS) was employed to determine the bulk elemental composition of the brackets before and after mechanical finishing. Unlike XPS, which is highly surface-sensitive, EDS collects signals from several micrometers beneath the surface and therefore represents the composition of the bulk material. Because mechanical finishing is a surface-level process, it is not expected to alter the underlying bulk chemistry. Nevertheless, EDS spectra were acquired for both the as-built and mechanically finished brackets to verify compositional consistency and confirm that no contamination or material loss occurred during processing. The front side of each bracket was analyzed, as there were no restrictions on sample mounting for this technique (Figure 7.8).

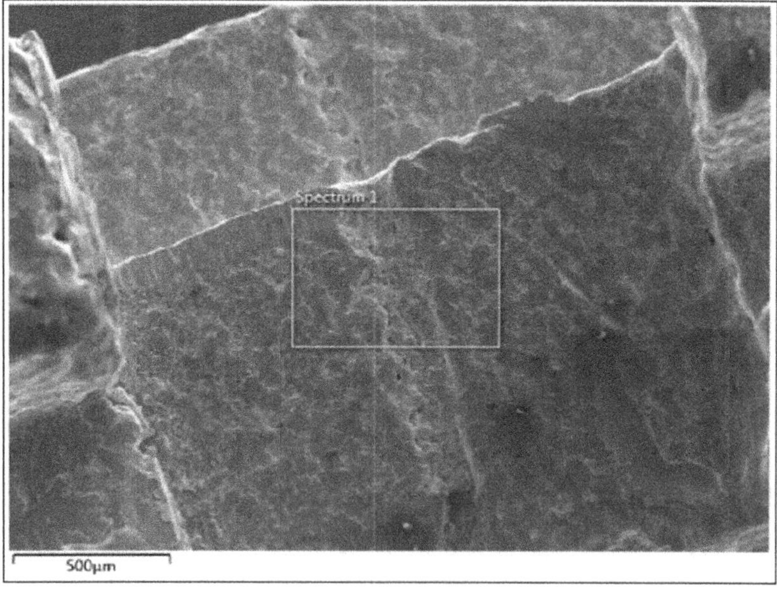

FIGURE 7.8   SEM image showing the front surface of the 3D-printed bracket.

The spectrum of the as-fabricated bracket (Figure 7.9) revealed iron (61.1 wt%) as the predominant element, followed by chromium (18.3 wt%) and nickel (11.2 wt%); minor alloying elements – aluminum (4.0 wt%), molybdenum (2.2 wt%), silicon (1.5 wt%), manganese (1.3 wt%), and titanium (0.3 wt%) – were also detected. Similarly, the finished bracket (Figure 7.10) displayed comparable bulk chemistry: iron (59.1 wt%), chromium (17.8 wt%), nickel (10.9 wt%), with minor components of aluminum (5.1 wt%), silicon (3.4 wt%), molybdenum (2.2 wt%), manganese (1.1 wt%), copper (0.3 wt%), and titanium (0.1 wt%). While the overall Fe–Cr–Ni balance reflects an austenitic stainless steel system, several measured elemental concentrations, particularly aluminum and silicon, do not fall within the compositional ranges specified for 316L stainless steel in ASTM A240/A240M–22 and ISO 5832-1:2016. Because both the as-built and rotary-finished brackets exhibited higher Al and Si levels, these anomalies are most likely linked to the experimental powder feedstock or to additive manufacturing artifacts such as oxide inclusions or spatter residues, rather than being introduced by finishing. Rotary tumbling may have further influenced the surface composition by embedding polishing media or altering the oxide layer, but it did not account for the initial presence of these elements. Furthermore, the brackets investigated here were experimental builds, and no certification was available to guarantee that the feedstock strictly met 316L stainless steel specifications. Accordingly, these results should be interpreted as surface-sensitive measurements rather than definitive evidence of bulk alloy deviation.

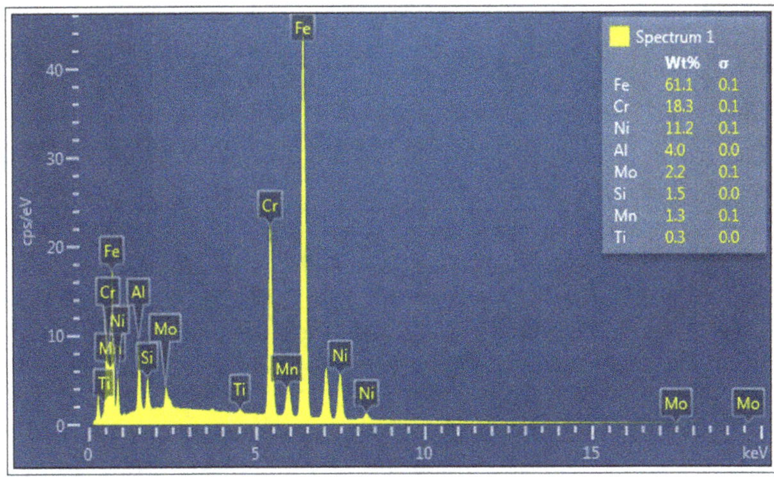

FIGURE 7.9 EDS spectrum of the as-built 3D-printed bracket.

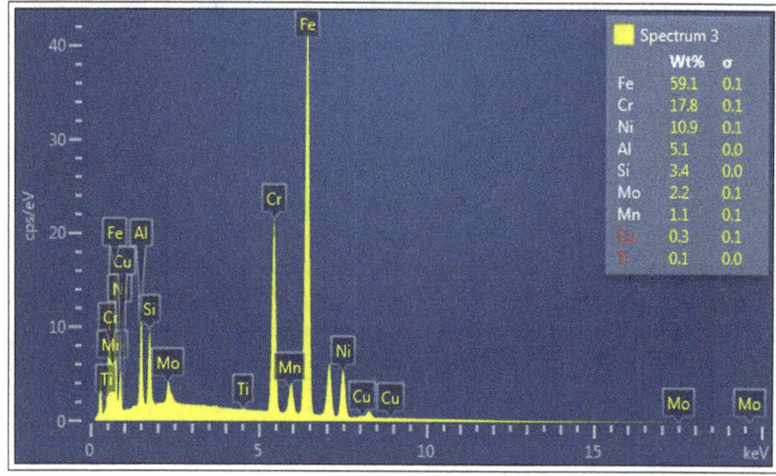

FIGURE 7.10   EDS spectrum of the mechanically finished 3D-printed bracket.

Summary of the Rotary Tumble Finishing

This section evaluated the rotary tumble finishing process for custom-made 3D-printed orthodontic brackets. Using silicon carbide abrasives in combination with ceramic pellets, the process achieved a 39% reduction in surface roughness. However, the observation of stained surface areas, which are potentially indicative of localized surface degradation, raises concerns regarding corrosion susceptibility. In its current form, rotary tumbling may therefore be unsuitable for clinical application, as orthodontic brackets must meet stringent biocompatibility requirements. Patients undergoing treatment must be assured of the long-term quality and safety of the brackets.

These observations, together with the findings from the literature review, support the idea that corrosion may develop over time on the surface of 3D-printed stainless steel brackets due to continuous exposure to moisture, fluctuating pH, and chemically aggressive conditions in the oral environment. Notably, without the rotary finishing step, such vulnerable surface regions may not have been readily identified, as the as-built surfaces appeared visually intact.

Surface analysis by X-ray photoelectron spectroscopy revealed elevated carbon levels on both as-built and mechanically finished brackets, with higher carbon content detected after rotary finishing. The as-built surface exhibited very low detectable chromium, likely influenced by surface morphology and measurement sensitivity, and was consistent with altered near-surface chromium availability. Energy-dispersive X-ray spectroscopy confirmed that the bulk compositions of as-built and finished brackets were similar. Nevertheless, since corrosion behavior is governed primarily by surface chemistry, these findings emphasize that alternative finishing strategies should be explored to achieve a surface composition with sufficient free chromium to ensure long-term corrosion resistance.

REFERENCES

ASTM International. (2022). *ASTM A240/A240M-22: Standard specification for chromium and chromium-nickel stainless steel plate, sheet, and strip for pressure vessels and general applications*. ASTM International. www.astm.org

Boonruang, C., & Sanumang, W. (2021). Effect of nano-grain carbide formation on electrochemical behavior of 316L stainless steel. *Scientific Reports, 11*, 12602. https://doi.org/10.1038/s41598-021-91958-x

DelVecchio, E., Liu, T., Chang, Y.-T., Nie, Y., Eslami, M., & Charpagne, M. A. (2024). Metastable cellular structures govern localized corrosion initiation in additively manufactured 316L stainless steel. *npj Materials Degradation, 8*, 45. https://doi.org/10.1038/s41529-024-00464-8

Federation of European Producers of Abrasives. (2006a). *FEPA standard 42-1:2006: Grains of fused aluminium oxide, silicon carbide and other abrasive materials for bonded abrasives – Part 1: Macrogrits F4 to F220*. FEPA. Retrieved from www.fepa-abrasives.org

Federation of European Producers of Abrasives. (2006b). *FEPA standard 42-2:2006: Grains of fused aluminium oxide, silicon carbide and other abrasive materials for bonded abrasives – Part 2: Microgrits F230 to F1200, F1500 to F12000*. FEPA. Retrieved from www.fepa-abrasives.org

International Organization for Standardization. (2016). *ISO 5832-1:2016 – Implants for surgery – Metallic materials – Part 1: Wrought stainless steel*. ISO.

Ko, G., Kim, W., Kwon, K., & Lee, T.-K. (2021). The corrosion of stainless steel made by additive manufacturing: A review. *Metals, 11*(3), 516. https://doi.org/10.3390/met11030516

Laleh, M., Hughes, A. E., Xu, W., Haghdadi, N., Wang, K., Cizek, P., Gibson, I., & Tan, M. Y. (2019). On the unusual intergranular corrosion resistance of 316L stainless steel additively manufactured by selective laser melting. *Corrosion Science, 161*, 108189. https://doi.org/10.1016/j.corsci.2019.108189

Li, S.-X., He, Y.-N., Yu, S.-R., & Zhang, P.-Y. (2013). Evaluation of the effect of grain size on chromium carbide precipitation and intergranular corrosion of 316L stainless steel. *Corrosion Science, 66*, 211–216. https://doi.org/10.1016/j.corsci.2012.09.022

Melia, M. A., Duran, J. G., Koepke, J. R., Saiz, D. J., Jared, B. H., & Schindelholz, E. J. (2020). How build angle and post-processing impact roughness and corrosion of additively manufactured 316L stainless steel. *npj Materials Degradation, 4*, 21. https://doi.org/10.1038/s41529-020-00126-5

Prochaska, S., & Hildreth, O. (2022). Effect of chemically accelerated vibratory finishing on the corrosion behavior of laser powder bed fusion 316L stainless steel. *Journal of Materials Processing Technology, 305*, 117596. https://doi.org/10.1016/j.jmatprotec.2022.117596

Sangoi, K., Nadimi, M., Song, J., & Fu, Y. (2025). Heat treatment effect on the corrosion resistance of 316L stainless steel produced by laser powder bed fusion. *Metals, 15*(1), 41. https://doi.org/10.3390/met15010041

Sharretts Plating Company. (2023). *Rotary and vibratory finishing*. Retrieved from www.sharrettsplating.com

Tian, M., Choundraj, J. D., Voisin, T., Wang, Y. M., & Kacher, J. (2022). Discovering the nanoscale origins of localized corrosion in additive manufactured stainless steel 316L by liquid cell transmission electron microscope. *Corrosion Science, 208*, 110659. https://doi.org/10.1016/j.corsci.2022.110659

Case Study
Electropolishing of Additively Manufactured Orthodontic Brackets

8

The findings reported in the previous chapter indicated that rotary tumble finishing, while effective in reducing surface roughness, may compromise surface chemistry and, consequently, the biocompatibility of additively manufactured stainless steel orthodontic brackets. This outcome necessitated an investigation of an alternative finishing process capable of achieving the required smoothness without degrading corrosion resistance.

This chapter focuses on electropolishing, identified as a second feasible finishing technique for custom-made stainless steel orthodontic brackets. The chapter presents: (i) a description of the electropolishing process and its operating principles, (ii) variation of key input parameters, (iii) characterization of samples before and after processing, (iv) quantitative evaluation of the finishing outcomes, and (v) surface and bulk chemical analyses. As in Chapter 7, the evaluation of key performance parameters employs the surface characterization methodologies previously described.

DOI: 10.1201/9781003772897-9

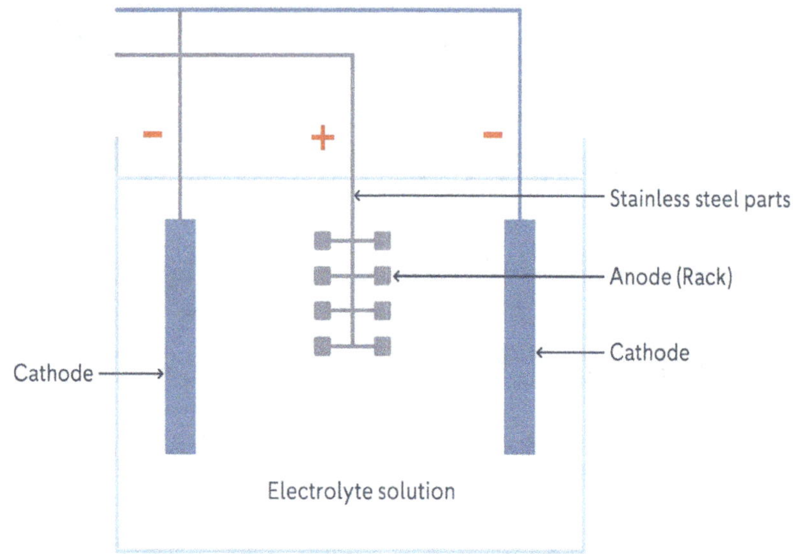

FIGURE 8.1   General schematic of the electropolishing process.

PROCESS OVERVIEW

Electrochemical etching, also referred to as electropolishing, electrochemical polishing, or electrolytic etching, represents a finishing process used to improve key performance parameters of high-quality brackets, including inherent corrosion resistance and surface smoothness. Figure 8.1 illustrates the general scheme of the electropolishing process.

In this process, material is removed ion-by-ion as the workpiece (anode) is immersed in an electrolyte solution and subjected to direct current flow toward a cathode. Due to differences in ohmic resistance between surface peaks and valleys, prominent asperities dissolve more rapidly than recessed areas, leading to progressive surface leveling (Landolt, 1987; Tyagi et al., 2019). Hydrogen gas is generated at the cathode as a by-product of the reduction reaction.

The material removal rate can be described by Faraday's first law of electrolysis (Encyclopaedia Britannica, n.d.):

$$f_r = \frac{CI}{A},$$

(8.1)

where:

f_r [mm/s] – material removal rate (feed rate), C [mm³/A·s] – specific removal rate (material-dependent), I [A] – current between anode and cathode, and A [mm²] is the frontal cathode area projected toward the workpiece.

Given the applied voltage E [V] and using Ohm's law, $I = \dfrac{E}{R}$, and expressing resistance R as gr/A (where g [mm] is the inter-electrode gap and r [Ω·mm] is the electrolyte resistivity), the current can be rewritten as:

$$I = \frac{EA}{gr} \tag{8.2}$$

Substituting into the original expression yields:

$$f_r = \frac{CE}{gr} \tag{8.3}$$

The polishing depth, T, is then given by:

$$T = tf_r \tag{8.4}$$

where t [s] is the polishing time.

These equations demonstrate that polishing depth is controllable and can be precisely adjusted to meet dimensional and surface accuracy requirements.

Over the past decade, electropolishing has evolved from a general finishing method to a highly controlled process for advanced manufacturing applications. Early studies demonstrated that material removal in stainless steels during electropolishing can range from 3 μm to over 50–80 μm, depending on current density, polishing time, electrolyte temperature, and acid concentration (Landolt, 1987). More recent work has refined these parameters to achieve near-machined smoothness, enhanced corrosion behavior, and clinical suitability for medical-grade components (Gorey et al., 2023).

Electropolishing is widely recognized as an effective post-processing technique for additively manufactured stainless steels, providing simultaneous improvements in surface smoothness and corrosion resistance, often associated with enhanced stability and chromium enrichment of the passive oxide layer (Tyagi et al., 2019; Gorey et al., 2023). Building on this context, the present study applies electropolishing under a straightforward set of process conditions to evaluate its ability to reduce surface roughness and enhance corrosion resistance in AM stainless steel orthodontic brackets, thereby directly addressing the second hypothesis of this work.

ELECTROPOLISHING: CHARACTERIZATION OF AM BRACKETS

Electropolishing of the additively manufactured bracket samples was carried out using an electrolyte composed of nitric, sulfuric, and phosphoric acids. Each bracket was mounted on a titanium rack, serving as the anode, and immersed in the electrolyte bath. Stainless steel cathodes and a rectifier completed the direct current (DC) electropolishing cell. The two primary controllable parameters, such as applied DC current and processing time, were adjusted based on the surface roughness achieved during preliminary trials.

Figure 8.2 presents Hirox microscope images (50×) of three representative samples before and after electropolishing. Panels (a), (c), and (e) correspond to the as-built 3D printed brackets, while panels (b), (d), and (f) show the same samples following electropolishing.

Changes in surface appearance for the measured archwire and upper regions of the three samples are summarized in Table 8.1. These measurement areas correspond to those defined in Chapter 6 for the characterization of traditionally machined and as-built AM brackets, enabling direct comparison of results.

Figure 8.3 demonstrates microscope images of the defined areas with 350× magnification of three representative samples before and after electropolishing. Panels A and B correspond to the archwire and upper areas of the as-built 3D printed bracket (Sample 1); panels C, E, and G show the archwire area of the electropolished samples (Samples 1, 2, and 3, respectively), and D, F, and H demonstrate their upper area.

DISCUSSION OF SURFACE ROUGHNESS RESULTS

As shown in Table 8.2, electropolishing generally reduced the surface roughness of the AM stainless steel brackets compared to their initial states. The most significant improvement was achieved for Sample 3, where the average Ra decreased from 5.28 μm to 2.59 μm after processing at 8.5 V for 4 minutes, representing the smoothest finish among all tested samples. According to Figure 8.4, which illustrates the surface roughness trend, higher voltage combined with adequate polishing time can effectively remove

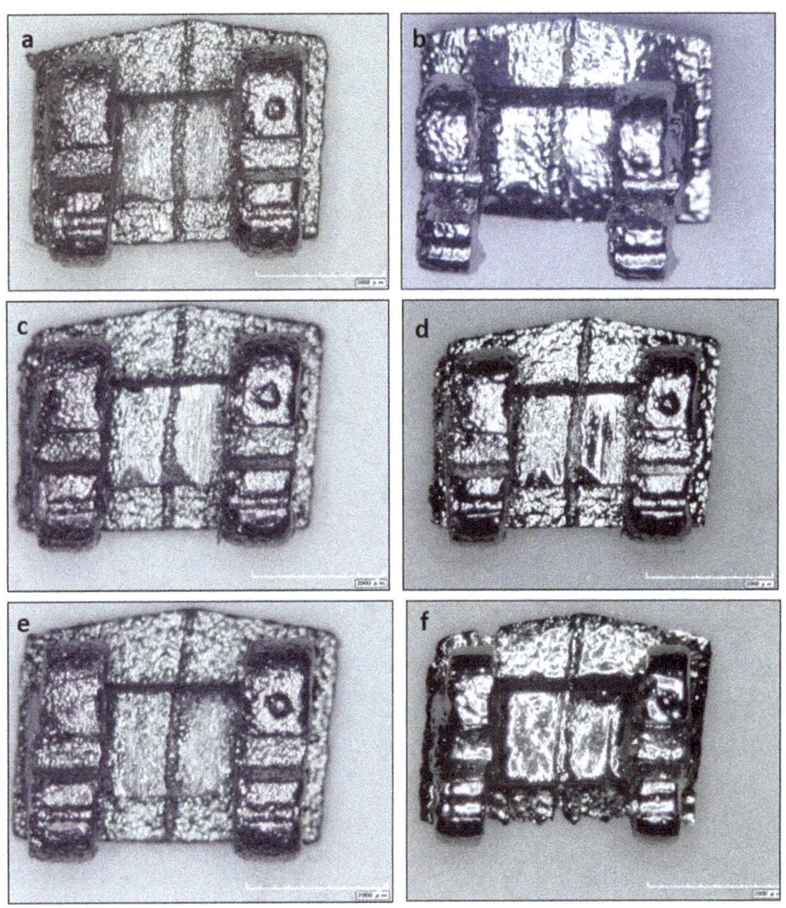

FIGURE 8.2   Hirox microscope images (50×) of 3D-printed brackets before and after electropolishing: a,b) Sample 1; c,d) Sample 2; e,f) Sample 3.

micro-asperities and yield a more uniform surface. By contrast, Sample 1 experienced an increase in Ra, likely due to residual microscopic peaks caused by insufficient treatment time. These results confirm that both applied voltage and duration must be carefully balanced to achieve optimal surface finish through electropolishing.

Visual inspection of the microscope images in Figures 8.2 and 8.3 supports these findings, with electropolished surfaces appearing brighter and smoother, suggesting improved topography and potential enhancement of corrosion resistance.

TABLE 8.1 Surface appearance changes in AM brackets before and after electropolishing (observed by Hirox microscope)[1]

SAMPLE NO.	ELECTROPOLISHING PARAMETERS	REGION	INITIAL SURFACE APPEARANCE	POST-ELECTROPOLISHING APPEARANCE
1	5 V, 2 min	Archwire	Pronounced ridges and irregular peaks	Noticeably smoother, rounded peaks
	5 V, 2 min	Upper	Uneven texture with visible adhered particles	Flattened texture, reduced debris
2	3 V, 3 min	Archwire	Clear layering and sharp asperities	Smoother profile, less pronounced steps
	3 V, 3 min	Upper	Irregular surface with minor porosity	More uniform texture, reduced porosity
3	8.5 V, 4 min	Archwire	Distinct striations and elevated ridges	Significantly reduced ridges, improved uniformity
	8.5 V, 4 min	Upper	Coarse topography with visible layer lines	Considerably smoother surface, layer lines largely diminished

1 The qualitative descriptions are based on Hirox microscope images; corresponding micrographs are shown in Figure 8.2b, d, f (50×) and Figure 8.3a-h (350×).

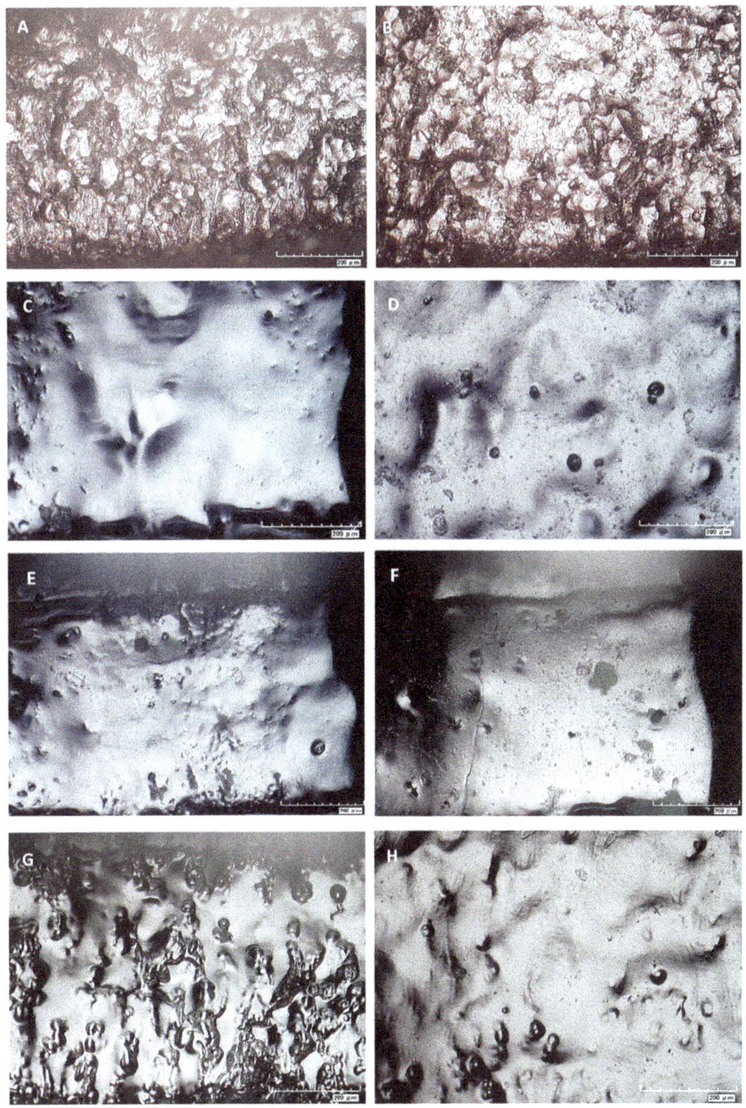

FIGURE 8.3 Hirox microscope images (350x) of 3D-printed brackets before and after electropolishing: (A, B) As-printed AM bracket: archwire (A), upper area (B), (C-H) Electropolished brackets: archwire area (C, E, G) and upper area (D, F, H) for Sample 1, Sample 2, Sample 3, respectively[a].

a The original (as-printed) views are shown only for Sample 1 (panels A, B), as the initial surfaces of Samples 2 and 3 were nearly identical to Sample 1; this was done to streamline the figure and present a concise visual comparison.

TABLE 8.2   Surface Roughness (R_a) of AM stainless steel brackets before and after electropolishing

| SAMPLE № | MEASURED PART | SURFACE ROUGHNESS R_A (μm) | | | | |
| | | ARCHWIRE AREA | | UPPER AREA | | |
		ALONG X	ALONG Y	ALONG X	ALONG Y	AVERAGE R_A
Sample 1	Initial part	89	4.85	3.74	4.68	4.92
	Electropolished (5 V, 2 min)	9.0	14.5	5.66	4.24	8.35
Sample 2	Initial part	7.34	6.91	3.17	3.13	5.14
	Electropolished (3 V, 3 min)	5.27	4.07	2.76	3.06	3.79
Sample 3	Initial part	9.58	4.85	2.48	4.21	5.28
	Electropolished (8.5 V, 4 min)	1.76	4.31	2.23	2.06	2.59

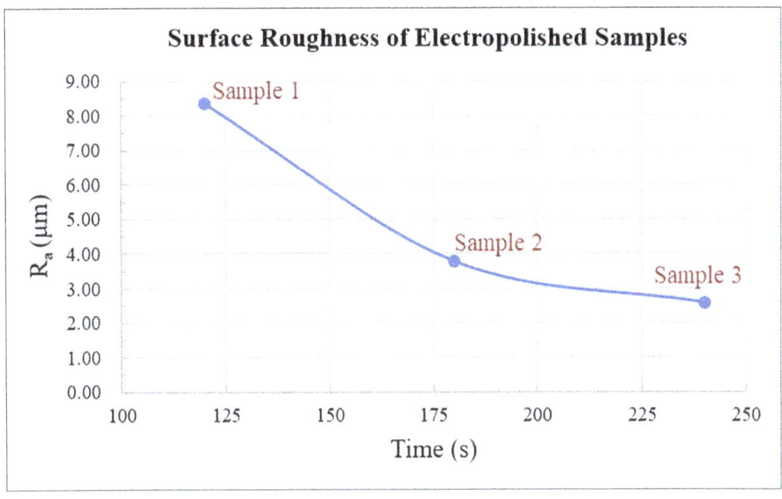

FIGURE 8.4   Variation of surface roughness (Ra) with finishing time.

Building on these surface quality findings, the following section examines how electropolishing influenced bracket geometry, assessing dimensional changes that could affect mechanical performance and fit in with orthodontic applications.

BRACKET GEOMETRY CHANGE AFTER ELECTROPOLISHING

During electropolishing, a certain amount of material is removed in accordance with Equation (8.4); therefore, dimensional changes must be considered. Table 8.3 presents measurements of the original and electropolished parts, obtained using the same 50× microscope. The column "Dimensional change Δ" represents the amount of material removed.

According to Table 8.3, electropolishing removed between 49 µm and 308 µm from the bracket surfaces. The amount of dissolved metal depends on process parameters such as voltage and polishing time, as described in Equations (8.3) and (8.4). For example, Sample 2, processed at 3 V for 3 min, lost only 49–59 µm, while Sample 3, processed at 8.5 V for 4 min, lost 298–308 µm.

TABLE 8.3   Dimensional measurements of the initial and finished brackets

SAMPLE	DIRECTION	INITIAL DIMENSION (I) (μm)	FINISHED DIMENSION (F) (μm)	DIMENSIONAL CHANGE $\Delta = I - F$ (μm)
1	Horizontal	4433	4286	147
	Vertical	3271	3112	159
2	Horizontal	4484	4425	59
	Vertical	3258	3209	49
3	Horizontal	4425	4127	298
	Vertical	3255	2947	308

Since Sample 3 achieved the lowest surface roughness, its metal removal rate was calculated using Equation (8.4). Assuming horizontal and vertical directions as "directional," the rates were:

$$f_{r\ horizontal} = 1.24*10^{-3} \text{mm/sec},$$

$$f_{r\ vertical} = = 1.28*10^{-3} \text{mm/sec}.$$

Electropolishing time and removed thickness showed a linear relationship (Figure 8.5).

To maintain required dimensions after post-processing, material removal should be accounted for in the CAD design of AM brackets. Equation (8.5) provides the adjustment:

$$Initial\ Directional\ Size + Directional\ Size\ Delta =$$
$$= Required\ Directional\ Size \qquad (8.5)$$

Using Sample 3 data from Table 8.3, the adjusted design dimensions are given in Table 8.4.

Based on these results, for electropolishing at 8.5 V and 4 min, the initial CAD model should include an additional 298 μm in the horizontal dimension and 308 μm in the vertical dimension. This pre-compensation allows for achieving the target final geometry after electropolishing without altering the functional design of the bracket.

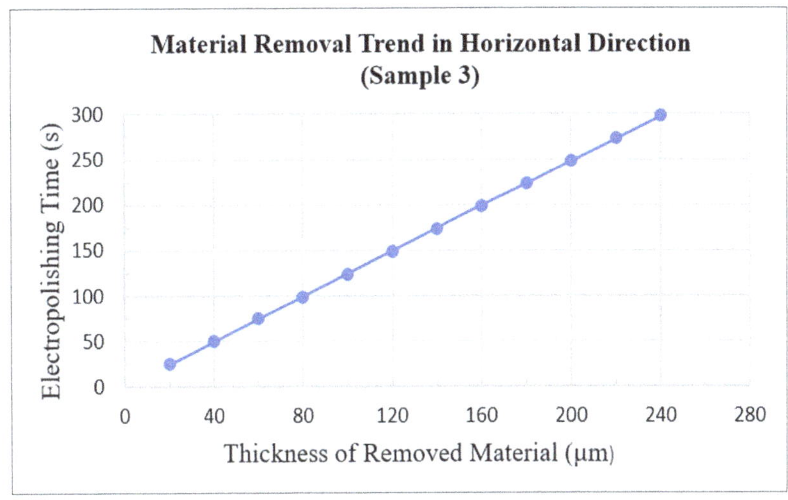

FIGURE 8.5 Material removal trend for Sample 3 during electropolishing.

SURFACE CHARACTERIZATION BY X-RAY PHOTOELECTRON SPECTROSCOPY (XPS)

XPS analysis was performed on the electropolished AM stainless steel bracket following the same procedure as for the as-built and mechanically finished parts: the sample was cleaned with an alcohol solution, and the back side of the bracket was used for measurement to avoid archwire slot interference.

The resulting spectrum (Figure 8.6) revealed major surface components: carbon (47.7 at%), oxygen (45.0 at%), chromium (1.5 at%), and other metallic elements, including phosphorus (5.8 at%). The quantitative comparison of surface elemental composition for the as-built and electropolished brackets is summarized in Table 8.5.

Compared with the as-built bracket, the electropolished surface exhibited a substantially lower carbon content and a higher oxygen concentration, consistent with the removal of carbon-rich surface layers and the development of a more oxidized passive film. Binding energy analysis indicated the presence of chromium oxide species on the bracket surface in both conditions; however, electropolishing increased the surface oxygen content ($\approx$30.8 to $\approx$45 at%) and produced a modest increase in the detected chromium signal ($\approx$1.1 to $\approx$1.5 at%), suggesting enrichment and/or thickening of the chromium-containing

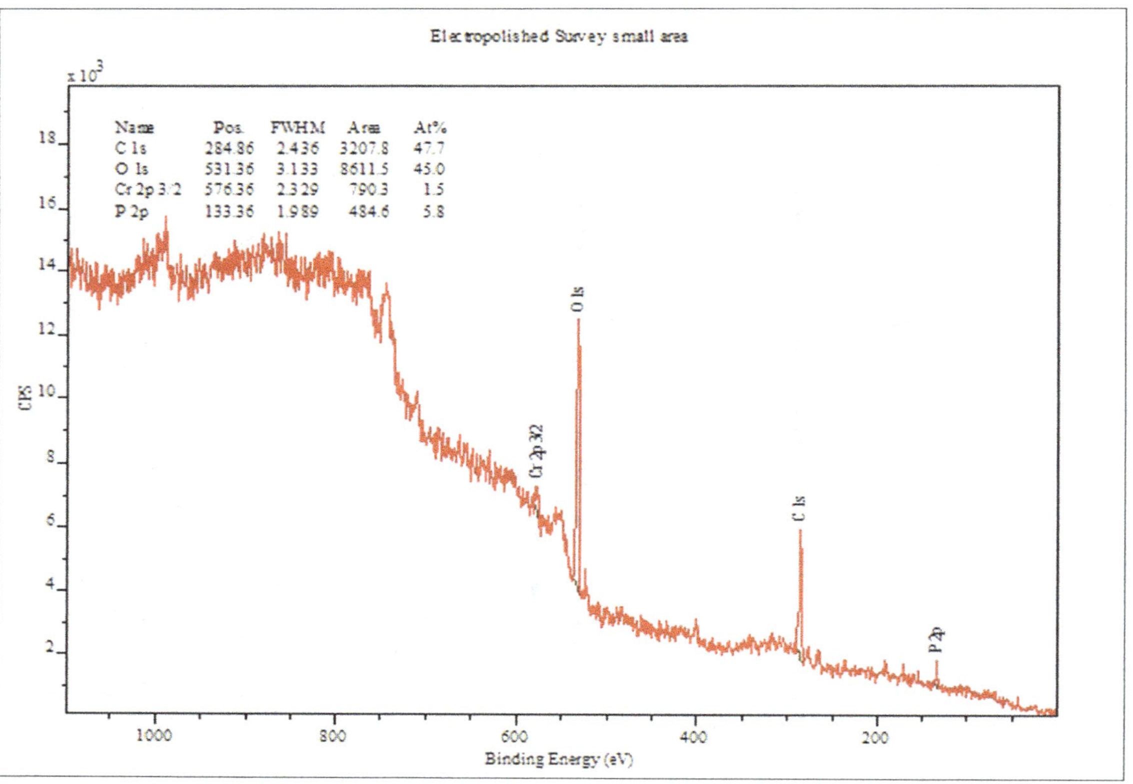

FIGURE 8.6   XPS spectrum of the electropolished 3D-printed bracket surface.

TABLE 8.4 Adjusted dimensions for Sample 3 based on material removal

DIRECTION	INITIAL (μm)	Δ (μm)	REQUIRED SIZE (μm)
Horizontal	4425	298	4723
Vertical	3255	308	3563

TABLE 8.5 Surface elemental composition (at%) of as-built and electropolished AM stainless steel brackets obtained by XPS

	ELEMENT	AS-BUILT AM BRACKET (AT%)	ELECTROPOLISHED AM BRACKET (AT%)
1	Carbon (C)	68.2	47.7
2	Oxygen (O)	30.8	45.0
3	Chromium (Cr)	1.1	1.5
4	Metals (Others)	ND	5.8

passive oxide layer. Chromium-rich oxides are widely recognized for their role in stabilizing passivity and enhancing corrosion resistance in stainless steels (Hryniewicz et al., 2009). Trace phosphorus detected on the electropolished surface is likely attributable to residual electrolyte species, a phenomenon reported in prior electropolishing studies (Rokosz et al., 2015). Such residues may be minimized through optimization of bath temperature and post-processing rinsing protocols, although corresponding adjustments to applied voltage and polishing time would be required.

SURFACE CHARACTERIZATION BY ENERGY-DISPERSIVE X-RAY SPECTROSCOPY (EDS)

EDS was used to determine the bulk elemental composition of the third electropolished bracket. The analysis was performed on the front side of the sample, using the same procedure applied to the as-built and mechanically finished parts described in the previous chapter. The resulting spectrum (Figure 8.7) revealed the following composition (in wt%): iron (64.3), chromium (18.7), nickel (12.3) as the principal constituents, with molybdenum (2.6), and minor amounts of manganese (1.0), silicon (0.7), and aluminum

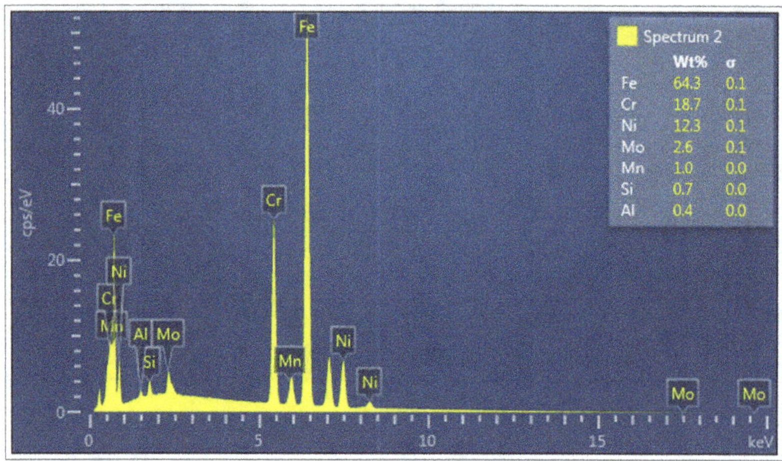

FIGURE 8.7   EDS spectrum of the electropolished 3D-printed bracket.

(0.4). The concentrations of the major alloying elements (Fe–Cr–Ni–Mo) are consistent with the nominal composition of austenitic stainless steel 316L as defined in both ISO 5832-1:2016 and ASTM A240/A240-22. The presence of minor elements is attributed to feedstock variability or AM-related artifacts and does not indicate a deviation from the base alloy system. This interpretation is consistent with findings from other electropolishing studies on AM 316L, in which X-ray photoelectron spectroscopy has demonstrated chromium oxide enrichment and reduced surface carbon following electropolishing, while bulk alloy composition remains unchanged (Hryniewicz et al., 2009; Rokosz et al., 2015).

SUMMARY OF THE ELECTROPOLISHING PROCESS

This chapter examined electropolishing as a post-processing method for additively manufactured orthodontic brackets, focusing on its ability to modify near-surface chemistry while simultaneously improving surface topography. Results from three processed samples demonstrated a marked improvement in surface smoothness and visual brightness relative to the as-printed condition. As noted by Tyagi et al. (2020), surface brightness and smoothness are widely used indicators of successful electropolishing, reflecting effective asperity leveling and surface conditions commonly associated with enhanced passivity and corrosion resistance.

X-ray photoelectron spectroscopy revealed a substantial reduction in surface carbon content following electropolishing, accompanied by a pronounced increase in surface oxygen and a modest increase in detectable chromium. Binding energy analysis indicated the presence of chromium oxide species in both the as-built and electropolished conditions, with electropolishing consistent with enrichment and/or thickening of the chromium-containing passive oxide layer. Energy-dispersive X-ray spectroscopy confirmed that bulk elemental composition remained unchanged, with iron, chromium, and nickel as the principal constituents. Collectively, these findings indicate that electropolishing improves surface condition and passivation without altering bulk chemistry, supporting its suitability for producing corrosion-resistant and biocompatible orthodontic bracket surfaces.

REFERENCES

ASTM International. (2022). *ASTM A240/A240M-22: Standard specification for chromium and chromium-nickel stainless steel plate, sheet, and strip for pressure vessels and general applications*. ASTM International. www.astm.org

Encyclopaedia Britannica (n.d.). *Faraday's laws of electrolysis*. Retrieved from www.britannica.com/science/Faradays-laws-of-electrolysis

Gorey, T. J., Stull, J. A., Hackenberg, R. E., Clark, C. L., & Hooks, D. E. (2023). Enhancing surface finish of additively manufactured 316L stainless steel with pulse/pulse reverse electropolishing. *JOM, 75*(6), 1728–1739. https://doi.org/10.1007/s11837-022-05558-9

Hryniewicz, T., Rokosz, K., & Filippi, M. (2009). Biomaterial studies on AISI 316L stainless steel after magnetoelectropolishing. *Materials, 2*(1), 129–145. https://doi.org/10.3390/ma2010129

International Organization for Standardization. (2016). *ISO 5832-1:2016 – Implants for surgery – Metallic materials – Part 1: Wrought stainless steel*. ISO.

Landolt, D. (1987). Fundamental aspects of electropolishing. *Electrochimica Acta, 32*(1), 1–11. https://doi.org/10.1016/0013-4686(87)87001-9

Rokosz, K., Hryniewicz, T., & Rzadkiewicz, S. (2015). XPS depth profiling analysis of passive layers formed on 316L stainless steel after electropolishing in a magnetic field. *Surface and Coatings Technology, 276*, 516–520. https://doi.org/10.1016/j.surfcoat.2015.06.022

Tyagi, P., Brent, D., Saunders, T.,Goulet, T., Riso, C., Klein, K., & García-Moreno, F. (2020). Roughness reduction of additively manufactured steel by electropolishing. *International Journal of Advanced Manufacturing Technology*, 106, 1337–1344 (2020). https://doi.org/10.1007/s00170-019-04720-z

Tyagi, P., Goulet, T., Riso, C., Stephenson, R., Chuenprateep, N., Schlitzer, J., Benton, C., & Garcia-Moreno, F. (2019). Reducing the roughness of internal surface of an additive manufacturing produced 316 steel component by chempolishing and electropolishing. *Additive Manufacturing*, 25, 32–38. https://doi.org/10.1016/j.addma.2018.11.001

Case Study Results and Discussion

9

DISCUSSION OF ROTARY TUMBLE FINISHING RESULTS

Rotary tumble finishing was evaluated as a mechanical post-processing approach for additively manufactured (AM) stainless steel orthodontic brackets to assess whether surface roughness could be reduced to clinically relevant levels without adversely affecting surface chemistry (Hypothesis 1).

The process employed silicon carbide and aluminum oxide abrasives, selected for their high hardness relative to stainless steel and common use in medical device finishing. Due to the complex geometry of orthodontic brackets, a range of abrasive grit sizes was required to promote contact with both external and internal features. Coarse grits (F60/90 and F150/220) produced limited net improvement in surface quality, likely because material removal at asperity peaks was accompanied by the introduction of new surface scratches, particularly along the build direction. The most effective results were achieved using F500 and F8000 grit in aqueous suspension, reducing the average surface roughness from 4.19 µm to 2.56 µm (39% reduction) after a cumulative processing time of 237 hours. This value approached the surface roughness of conventionally machined brackets (2.02 µm).

Despite this improvement in surface topography, X-ray photoelectron spectroscopy (XPS) indicated notable changes in near-surface chemistry

DOI: 10.1201/9781003772897-10

following mechanical finishing. Compared with the as-built condition, the mechanically finished surfaces exhibited increased surface carbon content and reduced oxygen concentration, suggesting modification of the native passive film and/or adsorption of carbon-rich surface species. High carbon content in austenitic stainless steels is undesirable because it can promote chromium carbide precipitation, resulting in localized chromium depletion along grain boundaries and reduced corrosion resistance (Hall & Briant, 1984; Ko et al., 2021).

Accordingly, while rotary tumble finishing proved effective in reducing surface roughness, it did not fully satisfy Hypothesis 1, as the observed changes in surface chemistry raise concerns regarding corrosion resistance and long-term biocompatibility.

DISCUSSION OF ELECTROPOLISHING RESULTS

Electropolishing was examined as an alternative surface finishing process with the potential to enhance both surface topography and chemical stability (Hypothesis 2). Using optimized parameters of 8.5 V and 4 minutes of processing time, surface roughness was reduced from 5.28 μm to 2.59 μm, representing a 50% improvement (Table 9.1). This final Ra value is comparable to conventionally machined brackets and was accompanied by a visibly smoother, brighter surface (Chapter 8, Figures 8.2–8.3).

XPS analysis of the electropolished surface revealed a substantial reduction in surface carbon content (47.7 at%) and increased oxygen (45.0 at%) and chromium (1.5 at%) levels compared to both the as-built and mechanically finished parts (Table 9.2). The elevated oxygen content is consistent with the presence of chromium-containing oxide species associated with passive film formation and enhanced corrosion resistance. The detection of phosphorus is

TABLE 9.1   Surface roughness results of finished 3D-printed and conventional brackets

	INITIAL R_A (μm)	FINAL R_A (μm)	IMPROVEMENT (%)
Conventional	2.02	-	-
Mechanical finishing	4.19	2.56	39
Electropolishing	5.28	2.59	50

TABLE 9.2 XPS elemental composition (at%) of AM stainless steel brackets

ELEMENT	ORIGINAL SAMPLE (AT%)	MECHANICAL FINISHING (AT%)	ELECTROPOLISHING (AT%)
Carbon	68.2	78.7	47.7
Oxygen	30.8	21.3	45.0
Chromium	1.1	-	1.5
Phosphorous	-	-	5.8

most likely attributed to electrolyte residues, which could be mitigated by additional rinsing or adjusting bath temperature.

Dimensional analysis revealed that electropolishing removed 298 μm (horizontal) and 308 μm (vertical) from the bracket (Sample 3). To maintain dimensional accuracy in clinical applications, these values should be incorporated into the initial CAD design of AM brackets.

Electropolishing satisfied Hypothesis 2 by achieving substantial surface roughness reduction while improving surface chemistry, resulting in a surface more resistant to corrosion and suitable for intraoral use.

DISCUSSION OF EDS RESULTS

Energy-dispersive X-ray spectroscopy (EDS) was employed to assess the elemental composition of brackets across three processing conditions: as-fabricated, mechanically finished, and electropolished. In all cases, iron, chromium, and nickel were the principal constituents, confirming an austenitic stainless steel system consistent with 300-series alloys.

Both the as-built and mechanically finished (rotary tumbled) samples exhibited elevated aluminum and silicon contents relative to the nominal composition of 316L stainless steel. Because these elements are not intentional alloying constituents, their detection is most likely attributed to the experimental feedstock variability or to surface-level artifacts inherent to SEM-EDS, such as oxide films, spatter residues, or nonmetallic inclusions. The persistence of Al and Si across both conditions indicates that these anomalies were present from the start and not introduced by finishing. In addition, the surface roughness and possible embedding of tumbling media may have further exaggerated these apparent deviations.

By contrast, the electropolished specimen yielded values that closely matched the compositional ranges defined for 316L stainless steel in both

ASTM A240/A240M–22 and ISO 5832-1:2016. This alignment supports the interpretation that electropolishing removed surface contaminants and mechanically altered layers, revealing a bulk composition consistent with the intended alloy.

Collectively, the EDS results demonstrate that finishing methods can influence apparent elemental composition because of surface effects and measurement sensitivity, but they do not fundamentally change the alloy chemistry. The electropolished condition provided the most reliable confirmation of 316L compliance, whereas differences observed by XPS in this study primarily reflect surface chemical modifications of the passive oxide film rather than changes in bulk composition.

SUMMARY AND COMPARATIVE ASSESSMENT

While both methods reduced surface roughness, only electropolishing preserved and enhanced near-surface chemical characteristics consistent with improved corrosion performance, as evidenced by reduced surface carbon content, increased surface oxidation, and enrichment and/or thickening of the chromium-containing passive oxide layer. Accordingly, electropolishing is recommended for clinical applications, with appropriate design-stage compensation to account for material removal during processing.

IMPLICATIONS FOR HYPOTHESES

- Hypothesis 1 – *Rotary tumble finishing can produce a smooth surface topography on AM stainless steel brackets without compromising surface chemistry.*
  Partially supported. While rotary tumble finishing reduced surface roughness to values approaching those of conventionally manufactured brackets, XPS analysis revealed elevated surface carbon levels and reduced oxygen content, indicating potential disruption of surface passivation and increased susceptibility to corrosion.
- Hypothesis 2 – *Electropolishing can enhance both surface smoothness and chemical stability.*

Supported. Electropolishing achieved an approximately 50% reduction in surface roughness, promoted development of a chromium-containing passive oxide layer, and reduced surface carbon content. Collectively, these changes are consistent with enhanced surface passivation and improved corrosion performance.

REFERENCES

Hall, E. L., & Briant, C. L. (1984). Chromium depletion in the vicinity of carbides in sensitized austenitic stainless steels. *Metallurgical Transactions A, 15*(3), 793–811. https://doi.org/10.1007/BF02644554

Ko, G., Kim, W., Kwon, K., & Lee, T.-K. (2021). The corrosion of stainless steel made by additive manufacturing: A review. *Metals, 11*(3), 516. https://doi.org/10.3390/met11030516

Conclusions and Future Directions

10

Custom-made orthodontic brackets designed with patient-specific morphologies demonstrate clear advantages for improving the mechanical effectiveness of orthodontic treatment. In contrast, conventionally machined brackets lack the flexibility to adapt to individual tooth surfaces. However, if patients are presented with a traditional bracket and a non-finished custom-made bracket, most would likely choose the traditional version due to its smooth surface, reduced friction, and superior appearance. The as-printed roughness of additively manufactured brackets not only increases friction between the archwire and bracket, resulting in less efficient tooth movement and extended treatment times, but also provides favorable sites for bacterial colonization within the oral cavity.

This study explored post-processing methods of rotary tumble finishing and electropolishing to assess their ability to produce high-performance, biocompatible AM stainless steel brackets. The aim was to reduce surface roughness and improve corrosion resistance, thereby approaching the quality of conventionally manufactured brackets.

KEY FINDINGS

- Rotary Tumble Finishing reduced surface roughness of 3D printed stainless steel brackets by 39%, from an initial Ra=4.19 μm to Ra=2.56 μm, with silicon carbide F500 and aluminum oxide F8000 proving the most effective media. This outcome brought the roughness close to that of conventionally machined brackets (Ra=2.02 μm), confirming the first hypothesis. However, surface

DOI: 10.1201/9781003772897-11

staining was observed post-finishing, potentially indicating localized corrosion initiation as per the literature review. XPS analysis revealed significant carbon presence, suggesting either contamination or non-passivated surfaces. Literature indicates that carbon is undesirable in austenitic stainless steels due to its affinity for chromium at elevated temperatures, further underscoring the need for chemical modification to ensure biocompatibility.

- Electropolishing achieved a substantial reduction in surface roughness, decreasing Ra by approximately 50% from 5.28 µm to 2.59 µm, and produced a smooth, bright surface finish. The electropolished samples exhibited markedly improved surface quality, which is expected to reduce bracket-archwire friction and support more physiologic tooth movement under clinical conditions. XPS analysis indicated the presence of chromium-containing oxide species on the electropolished surfaces, consistent with enhanced surface passivation and improved corrosion performance. Energy-dispersive X-ray spectroscopy confirmed that the bulk composition of all samples remained consistent with 300-series austenitic stainless steels; however, electropolishing resulted in the most chemically stable and passivated surface condition of the two finishing methods evaluated.

CONCLUSIONS

Taken together, these results demonstrate that electropolished AM stainless steel brackets meet the essential requirements for clinical application, including:

- Smooth and visually uniform surfaces,
- Surface roughness values approaching those of conventional brackets,
- Surface chemical conditions consistent with enhanced corrosion resistance through development of a passive oxide film.

Electropolishing therefore emerges as the most reliable and clinically feasible finishing technique for AM orthodontic brackets. Importantly, electropolishing is a parameter-dependent process, and its effectiveness is governed by the applied voltage, electrolyte composition, temperature, and processing time. Appropriate selection and control of these parameters are necessary to achieve optimal surface smoothing while preserving dimensional accuracy and surface chemistry.

When properly optimized, electropolished AM brackets can serve as biocompatible alternatives to conventional brackets, offering the additional advantages of design flexibility and cost efficiency inherent to additive manufacturing. Although the present findings demonstrate strong performance, further research is warranted to refine process windows, assess long-term clinical behavior, and establish standardized electropolishing protocols for orthodontic applications.

FUTURE RESEARCH DIRECTIONS FOR ADDITIVELY MANUFACTURED ORTHODONTIC BRACKETS

Additive manufacturing (AM) opens the door to orthodontic brackets that extend far beyond conventional geometric limitations. Future advances will integrate artificial intelligence, nanomaterials, biosurface engineering, and sensor technologies to produce devices that are not only customized but biologically and digitally responsive. The following directions illustrate where AM orthodontics is likely to evolve as the field matures.

♣ *AI-Driven Bracket Design*

One of the most transformative areas of future development is the application of artificial intelligence to individualized bracket design. Today's digital orthodontic workflows already incorporate patient-specific modeling, yet they remain largely dependent on manual prescription of torque, angulation, and offset. Machine-learning (ML) systems have begun to demonstrate their capacity to assist orthodontic treatment planning by predicting clinical decisions such as tooth extraction from diagnostic data, and emerging work suggests broader potential for ML to inform biomechanical understanding and personalized tooth movement forecasts (Huang et al., 2024). As these computational models evolve, they may become capable of generating bracket geometries autonomously, optimizing torque expression and force systems based on anatomical features, bone density distribution, and projected biological response.

This vision anticipates a workflow in which the clinician defines overarching treatment goals, while AI algorithms iteratively compute bracket geometry, simulate mechanical performance, and refine the design until biomechanical criteria are met. The manufacturing flexibility inherent to AM enables each bracket to be produced with a unique geometry without the cost constraints of traditional fabrication. AI-driven design paired with AM's geometric freedom could therefore yield orthodontic appliances with unprecedented precision and predictability.

♣ *Surface Engineering and Advanced Antimicrobial Nanocoatings*

Surface engineering represents another promising frontier for future AM brackets. Although electropolishing significantly improves surface smoothness and corrosion resistance, long-term performance in the biologically active oral environment may require more specialized interventions. Nanostructured antimicrobial coatings are of particular interest because they can reduce bacterial adhesion, stabilize the passive film, and mitigate plaque accumulation at a molecular level.

Titanium dioxide coatings, for example, have shown strong inhibitory activity against *Streptococcus mutans* and related oral bacteria via photocatalytic mechanisms that disrupt biofilm formation and bacterial physiology (Sanders et al., 2023). Graphene-based films similarly demonstrate potent antibacterial behavior through electron-transfer interactions and mechanical disruption of cell membranes (Li et al., 2014). These technologies may be integrated with electropolished AM surfaces to create durable, hygienic interfaces that maintain low roughness while resisting microbial colonization.

Future research will likely explore how such coatings interact with AM-specific surface features, whether they can withstand orthodontic loading and archwire engagement, and how they affect ion release and corrosion over the life of treatment. The convergence of surface finishing and nanomaterial engineering is expected to be instrumental in creating brackets that are not only mechanically effective but also biologically advantageous.

♣ *Sensor-Enabled "Smart Brackets"*

A third major direction involves the development of smart orthodontic brackets with embedded sensing capabilities. Advances in micro-electromechanical systems (MEMS) and flexible micro-sensors have shown potential for measuring biomechanical forces in small-scale biomedical devices (Rajagopalan et al., 2010). Additive manufacturing could allow sensor channels or cavities to be incorporated directly into bracket geometries, enabling real-time detection of force magnitude, direction, wire–slot friction, and even temperature changes associated with patient compliance.

Such sensors may allow clinicians to monitor treatment progression remotely and adjust force delivery with far greater precision than periodic in-office evaluations permit. In the future, orthodontic systems may become semi-autonomous, using data from sensor-equipped brackets to trigger adaptive treatment plans or alert clinicians when forces deviate from therapeutic ranges.

Powering these devices remains a challenge, though potential methods include inductive charging, miniature batteries, or energy harvesting from mastication forces. Overall, smart bracket technology represents a convergence of AM's geometric flexibility with digital health innovation, offering a pathway to fully instrumented orthodontic biomechanics.

❖ *Bioactive Surface Functionalization*

An additional area of emerging interest involves the development of bioactive surfaces that contribute positively to the oral environment. Rather than being chemically inert, future AM brackets may be engineered to support a healthy microbiome, reduce inflammation, or promote enamel protection. Research in dental implants demonstrates that surface coatings such as chitosan, hydroxy-apatite, and calcium–phosphate films are widely investigated for their potential to reduce bacterial adhesion and enhance biological integration at implant surfaces (Zafar et al., 2020).

Applying similar strategies to orthodontic brackets could lead to appliances that help mitigate common treatment complications, such as white spot lesions or localized gingival irritation. Bioactive surfaces may be particularly useful when combined with AM's ability to produce finely controlled topographies and microstructures that guide cellular or microbiological behavior.

❖ *Next-Generation Finishing Technologies and Hybrid Surface Treatments*

Although electropolishing remains one of the most effective methods for refining AM stainless steel, the next stage of research will likely focus on hybrid approaches that further enhance surface quality. Recent work on laser–electrochemical hybrid polishing of SLM 316L stainless steel demonstrates that combining thermal surface reflow with electrochemical smoothing produces exceptionally low roughness values and superior wear resistance compared with either technique alone (Liu et al., 2024). These methods may be particularly beneficial for orthodontic brackets, whose intricate geometries and tight tolerances demand both precision and effective material removal.

The electropolishing case study provides an example of how advanced finishing processes can meaningfully influence corrosion performance and surface morphology. Building on such findings, future work should examine hybrid polishing methods, laser re-melting sequences, and chemically functionalized post-processing protocols, accompanied by long-term in vivo evaluations to understand their effects on plaque retention, ion release, and host tissue response.

Taken together, these research directions highlight a future in which AM orthodontic brackets evolve into fully integrated, multifunctional therapeutic tools. Advances in AI-driven design could optimize biomechanics with unprecedented precision; surface engineering and nanomaterials could ensure hygienic and stable interfaces; embedded sensors could provide real-time information about treatment forces; and bioactive surfaces could support oral health at the microbial level. As these innovations converge, orthodontic brackets may transition from static mechanical devices to adaptive, intelligent, and biologically aligned components of a comprehensive digital treatment ecosystem.

REFERENCES

Huang, J., Chan, I.-T., Wang, Z., Ding, X., Jin, Y., Yang, C., & Pan, Y. (2024). Evaluation of four machine learning methods in predicting orthodontic extraction decision from clinical examination data and analysis of feature contribution. *Frontiers in Bioengineering and Biotechnology, 12*, 1483230. https://doi.org/10.3389/fbioe.2024.1483230

Li, J., Wang, G., Zhu, H., Zhang, M., Zheng, X., Di, Z., Liu, X., & Wang, X. (2014). Antibacterial activity of large-area monolayer graphene film manipulated by charge transfer. *Scientific Reports, 4*, 4359. https://doi.org/10.1038/srep04359

Liu, J., Li, C., Yang, H., Liu, J., Wang, J., Deng, L., Fang, L., & Yang, C. (2024). Study on laser–electrochemical hybrid polishing of selective laser melted 316L stainless steel. *Micromachines, 15*(3), 374. https://doi.org/10.3390/mi15030374

Rajagopalan, J., Tofangchi, A., & Saif, M. T. A. (2010). Linear high-resolution BioMEMS force sensors with large measurement range. *Journal of Microelectromechanical Systems, 19*(6), 1380–1389. https://doi.org/10.1109/JMEMS.2010.2076780

Sanders, M. K., Duarte, S., Ayoub, H. M., Scully, A. C., Vinson, L. A., & Gregory, R. L. (2023). Effect of titanium dioxide on *Streptococcus mutans* biofilm. *Journal of Applied Biomaterials & Functional Materials, 21*, 131892. https://doi.org/10.1177/22808000221131892

Zafar, M. S., Fareed, M. A., Riaz, S., Latif, M., Habib, S. R., & Khurshid, Z. (2020). Customized therapeutic surface coatings for dental implants. *Coatings, 10*(6), 568. https://doi.org/10.3390/coatings10060568

Index